AFib Diet Cookbook
A Heart-Healthy Recipes Guide

AFib Diet Cookbook; A Heart-Healthy Recipes Guide

A Practical Guide for Cardiovascular Health, Obesity and Atrial Fibrillation Reversal, Sustainable Weight Loss, Heart Disease, Stroke, Fatigue and healthy living

Lilian Daniel

Copyright

Disclaimer

Table of Contents

Introduction

Welcome to my kitchen, where every recipe is a celebration of good health and vibrant living. In this my latest cookbook, "Afib Diet Cookbook: A Heart-Healthy Recipes Guide," I'm thrilled to share with you a collection of nourishing dishes designed to nourish both body and soul.

But before we began my dearie, you might think, why should this cookbook matter to me? Well, my loves, let me tell you why it's important for everyone, from our dearest seniors to the youngest among us, and even the little ones who dream of becoming kitchen maestros themselves. You see, in the heart of every home, there lies a treasure trove of stories waiting to be told. And what better way to nourish those tales than with dishes created with care and love?

If you have been in the kitchen as long as I have, you will know that the key to our very existence depends on what we eat and drink.

Living with atrial fibrillation (AFib) can present its challenges, but through the power of delicious, heart-healthy food, we can take control of our health and embrace a life of wellness.

This cookbook isn't just about recipes, it is a practical guide to transforming your relationship with food and reclaiming your vitality.

As we proceed, you will find not only nourishing recipes created and designed to support cardiovascular health and promote sustainable weight loss, but also personal insights and practical tips gleaned from my own experiences in the kitchen. From shortcuts and substitutions to moments of triumph and the occasional mishap, I'm here to share it all with you.

Because cooking isn't just about following instructions, it is about creating something beautiful and nourishing with your own two hands. Whether you're a seasoned home cook or just starting out on your culinary journey. You will discover a treasure trove of flavorful dishes carefully crafted to support cardiovascular health, reverse obesity, and promote sustainable weight loss. From vibrant salads bursting with fresh produce to hearty soups that warm the soul, and as well nourish our bodies with wholesome ingredients.

This Edition, is more than just a collection of recipes, it's a roadmap to a healthier, happier life. Alongside delicious dishes, you'll find invaluable tips and insights on managing AFib, reducing the risk of heart disease and stroke, combating fatigue, and embracing a lifestyle of wellness.

So, join me in the kitchen, together let's find a way to a better health and vitality. With a dash of creativity, a sprinkle of inspiration, and a whole lot of love, we'll discover the power of food to heal, nourish, and rejuvenate. But before we proceed, we must first know what we are up against. So, what is AFib?

In the rhythm of our hearts, there's a beat that's off-key, an irregular dance of the upper chambers known as atrial fibrillation, or afib. When this rhythm goes awry, the heart races faster than its usual tempo, causing an irregular heartbeat, or arrhythmia. Left unattended, this discordant melody can crescendo into serious complications like stroke and other heart-related issues.

But fear not, for the symphony of wellness conducts its own counterpoint, a healthy diet. Yes, what we eat can orchestrate harmony in the face of afib, orchestrating a symphony of nutrients to reduce symptoms and mitigate the risk of further heart conditions.

Calories and alcohol take center stage in this dietary drama. Many who dance to the rhythm of afib find themselves weighed down by excess pounds. Yet, shedding this weight can serve as a conductor's baton, helping to regain control over the arrhythmic beats of afib.

Afib, while not life-threatening on its own, can conduct its own suite of risks: strokes, blood clots, and congestive heart failure. Imagine the heart's upper chambers, the atria, in a tumultuous ballet, twirling chaotically out of sync with the lower chambers, the ventricles. While some may hear no discordant notes, others may sense a rapid, pounding rhythm, or feel faint from the dissonance.

These episodes of afib may come and go like fleeting melodies, or linger as persistent refrains. Though not fatal in itself, afib is a serious condition demanding proper treatment to keep the symphony of the heart in tune and prevent the risk of stroke.

Treatment often requires a multifaceted approach, from medicinal harmonies to therapeutic interventions that shock the heart back into rhythm or block those faulty signals.

Yet even within this symphony of heart rhythms, there may be a related variation known as atrial flutter, marching to a similar beat. Thus, the treatments for both afib and atrial flutter harmonize, guiding the heart's melody back to its rightful tempo and restoring the rhythm of life.

To understand why atrial fibrillation (AFib) happens, let's look at how a normal heart works. Your heart has four parts:

- The top parts are called atria.

- The bottom parts are called ventricles.

Inside the right atrium, there's a group of cells called the sinus node. This group sends signals that start each heartbeat. These signals move across the atria and then to a group of cells called the AV node, where they usually slow down. After that, the signals go to the ventricles.

In a healthy heart, this process works smoothly. Your heart usually beats between 60 to 100 times a minute when you're resting. A normal heartbeat starts with one electrical impulse from the sinus node, a tiny spot in the right atrium.

But with AFib, electrical impulses come from different spots in both atria. This can make the atria contract more than 400 times a minute. The ventricles can't keep up with this fast pace. They beat faster than they should, and they might not have enough time to fill with blood and pump it properly.

So, blood stays in the atria instead of moving into the ventricles and out to the body. This can lead to blood clots forming in the heart. These clots can travel from the heart to the bloodstream and even to the brain, which can cause a stroke.

Causes and Risk of AFib

The most common reasons why people get atrial fibrillation (AFib) are problems with the heart's structure, some of which includes;

- Being born with a heart problem, known as a congenital heart defect.

- Issues with the heart's natural pacemaker, called sick sinus syndrome.

- Having a sleep disorder called obstructive sleep apnea.

- Having a heart attack.

- Heart valve disease.

- High blood pressure.

- Lung diseases like pneumonia.

- Narrowed or blocked arteries, also called coronary artery disease.

- Thyroid problems like an overactive thyroid.

➢ Infections caused by viruses.

Some of us develop AFib without having any known heart disease or damage. Certain lifestyle habits can also bring on an episode of AFib. These include:

- ○ Drinking too much alcohol or caffeine.

- ○ Using illegal drugs.

- ○ Smoking or chewing tobacco.

- ○ Taking medications that contain stimulants, like some cold and allergy medicines we buy without a prescription.

Certain things that make us more likely to develop atrial fibrillation (AFib) and some main risk factors are;

I. **Age:** The older we get, the higher our risk of AFib becomes.

II. **Changes in body minerals:** Electrolytes like potassium, sodium, calcium, and magnesium help regulate your heartbeat. If these minerals are too high or too low, it can cause irregular heartbeats.

III. **Heart problems or heart surgery:** Conditions like coronary artery disease, heart valve issues, and congenital heart defects can increase your risk of AFib. Previous heart attacks or surgeries also raise the likelihood of developing AFib.

IV. **Obesity:** Being overweight increases your risk of AFib.

V. **Other health conditions:** Diabetes, chronic kidney disease, lung problems, and sleep apnea can all raise your risk of AFib.

After assessing a person's risk of stroke, the next important step in managing AFib is to slow down their resting heart rate to about 80 beats per minute. This can be done using medications.

The second step involves deciding whether to control the person's heart rhythm with antiarrhythmic medications or a medical procedure. For those who experience AFib all the time, a procedure called cardioversion (using electrical shock) may help restore a normal rhythm. Medications or catheter ablation can then be used to help maintain this normal rhythm.

Making healthy lifestyle choices can also play a big role in reducing the risk of heart disease and possibly preventing AFib.

In my services to individual with AFib, I discover some simple tips to keep your heart healthy:

- Control high blood pressure, high cholesterol, and diabetes.

- Avoid smoking or using tobacco.

- Eat a diet low in salt and saturated fat.

- Aim to exercise for at least 30 minutes a day on most days of the week, unless your healthcare team advises otherwise.

- Get enough sleep, adults should aim for 7 to 9 hours each night.

- Maintain a healthy weight.

- Find ways to reduce and manage stress in your life.

Now, with that being said, if you have AFib, it's important to know which foods and drinks to avoid. For instance, your doctor might suggest you cut back or skip alcohol because it can cause problems. Individuals with atrial fibrillation often take blood thinners to prevent blood clots. If you're on a blood thinner like warfarin (Jantoven), your doctor might advise you to limit leafy green vegetables, as they have vitamin K. Too much vitamin K can affect how warfarin works in your body.

Making healthy changes to your diet can improve your heart health, aim to eat a heart-healthy diet that includes:

- Fruits

- Vegetables

- Whole grains

- Low-fat or fat-free dairy products

- Proteins like lean meats, nuts, seeds, and beans

Also, try to avoid foods that are high in salt, added sugars, saturated fat, and trans-fat.

Obesity and AFib Dieting

More and more people are experiencing an abnormal heart rhythm, known as atrial fibrillation (AFib). While things like family history and aging can contribute to this condition, there's something you can control that might increase your chances of having AFib: your weight.

Whether you're already at risk for AFib or simply want to improve your overall health, here's what you should know. Around 7.2 million people across Europe have AFib. If you are one of them, it means your heart isn't receiving the correct electrical signals to regulate its contractions and relaxations. This leads to irregular beating in the upper chambers, causing your heart to pump blood less effectively than it should.

AFib can cause symptoms like weakness, shortness of breath, and heart palpitations, when it feels like your heart has skipped a beat. You might also experience a fluttering sensation or feel like your heart is racing or pounding. Additionally, AFib increases your risk of more serious health issues, such as stroke, kidney disease, and heart failure.

If you are obese, meaning your body mass index (BMI) is 30 or higher, you're twice as likely to have AFib. But there's hope, you can make a change. Losing extra weight can really make a difference. In one study, obese individuals who lost at least 10% of their body weight were 10 times less likely to experience this abnormal heartbeat again.

Carrying extra fat, especially around your waist, can directly impact your heart. Over time, it can build up in your arteries and harm your heart's left ventricle, its main pumping chamber. This makes it harder for your heart to fill up properly between beats. Being overweight also causes changes in your heart's electrical and chemical functions. It can increase inflammation in your body. Plus, obesity often comes with other health issues like high blood pressure, coronary artery disease (CAD), sleep apnea, and diabetes. Each of these conditions is also linked to a higher risk of AFib.

The higher your BMI, the greater your chances of having AFib. So, shedding those extra pounds not only benefits your overall health but can also lower your risk of developing this heart condition.

Sometimes, doctors can treat AFib with medications that reset your heart's rhythm. But if medicine isn't an option or doesn't work, surgery might be necessary. One common AFib treatment is called cardiac ablation. During this procedure, the doctor guides a long tube, called a catheter, through your blood vessels and up to your heart. Then, they use radio waves, heat, or extreme cold to destroy the damaged tissue causing your AFib.

While ablation can eliminate the need for long-term medication or surgical implants to correct your heartbeat, it might not be the best choice if you are obese. People with higher BMIs have a greater chance of AFib returning after ablation compared to those with normal BMIs. Even small increases in BMI can increase the risk. If your BMI is over 40, you are more likely to experience side effects from cardiac ablation.

So, what's the best course of action if you're obese and at risk of AFib? Experts suggest that weight loss is the key.

Reaching a healthy weight can also help you manage other health issues like high blood pressure, sleep apnea, diabetes, and high cholesterol. When these conditions are in check, your heart can function better as well.

Steps by Step Procedure in Reducing Obesity and AFib Control

First off, when you are dealing with AFib and carrying around some extra pounds, you're in for a double whammy of health trouble. But here's the good news: what you put on your plate can be your secret weapon in this battle.

When it comes to AFib, a healthy diet can be like armor for your heart. We're talking about loading up on fresh, wholesome foods that pack a punch of nutrients without weighing you down with excess calories. Think vibrant fruits, crisp veggies, and hearty whole grains. These bad boys not only fuel your body but also help keep your ticker ticking smoothly.

And let's not forget about the dreaded obesity monster lurking in the shadows. Tackling this beast head-on requires a strategic approach to eating. That means cutting back on the junk and doubling down on lean proteins, nuts, seeds, and beans. We're talking about foods that fill you up without piling on the pounds.

But here's the real kicker, it's not just about what you eat, it's also about how you eat it. Portion control is key, my friends. No need to go all "Hulk smash" on your plate, keep it civilized and savor each mouthful. So, if you're ready to show AFib and obesity who is the boss, start by transforming your diet into a powerhouse of health. It's time to take control of your health, one delicious bite at a time

I.   **Eat less and move more;** *Cut down on the number of calories you eat and drink, and increase your physical activity. Your doctor can guide you on how to do this safely.*

II.   **Focus on healthy foods**; *Opt for fresh, whole foods like fruits, vegetables, and whole grains, which provide your body with essential nutrients without packing on extra calories.*

III.   **Start with small goals;** *Set clear and achievable goals that you're more likely to stick to. For example, commit to cooking a healthy dinner and skipping fast food two nights a week.*

IV.   **Keep track of your progress;** *Keep a food journal, count your steps, and regularly check in with a friend or counselor for support and accountability.*

V.   **Be patient;** *Weight loss takes time, sometimes months or even years, not days. Aim for sustainable lifestyle changes rather than quick-fix diets that leave you feeling deprived.*

Diet plays a big role in managing AFib by lowering the risk factors that cause it and sometimes easing its symptoms. A heart-healthy diet focuses on foods like fruits, vegetables, whole grains, and extra virgin olive oil, all of which are great for your heart and can help with AFib.

Like I said earlier on, this book is more than just a cookbook, let's take a closer look at the benefits of plant-based diets, whole grains, and extra virgin olive oil, giving you the best chance of managing AFib effectively.

PLANTS-BASED DIETS

Eating more plants is great for your heart! Plant-based diets give your body all the important nutrients it needs and can help lower inflammation. They're linked to a lower risk of diseases like heart disease and type 2 diabetes, and they can even improve how well your kidneys work.

So, what should you eat? Load up on fruits, veggies, beans, fish, nuts, and olive oil, these are all key parts of diets which are especially good for managing AFib.

A plant-based diet full of fruits, veggies, and healthy fats can boost your heart health overall, lower your cholesterol, and reduce your risk of a heart attack. Making the switch to a plant-based diet is a proactive move to better manage your AFib and keep your heart in top shape.

The Importance of Whole Grain

Whole grains are super important for a healthy heart. They are packed with fiber, vitamins, minerals, and antioxidants, all of which are great for your cardiovascular health. Eating whole grains has been related to better heart health, improved control of blood sugar levels, and easier weight management.

Some examples of whole grains include brown rice, oats, quinoa, and barley. By adding these grains to your diet, you're not only boosting your heart health, but also helping to keep your blood sugar levels in check and manage your weight. And all of these things can help lower your chances of developing AFib.

Benefits of Extra Virgin Olive Oil

Extra virgin olive oil is like liquid gold for your heart. It is a key part of a heart-healthy diet and can-do wonders for preventing AFib. This magical oil is packed with anti-inflammatory and antioxidant powers, which can help lower your risk of heart disease.

In fact, a study called the PREDIMED trial found that adding extra virgin olive oil to your diet can slash your risk of AFib by a whopping 38%! So, by drizzling some of this oil onto your meals, you're not only making them taste delicious, but you're also reaping the benefits for your heart.

Some of the perks of extra virgin olive oil include;

- Reducing inflammation

- Fighting off harmful oxidative stress

- Supporting heart health

- Lowering blood pressure

- Improving cholesterol levels.

With all these amazing benefits, it's no wonder this oil is a superstar in any heart-healthy and AFib-friendly diet.

Now, let's talk about the foods you should be including in your AFib diet. You will want to focus on foods that are high in fiber, lean proteins, and packed with antioxidants. These goodies will help keep your heart happy and your AFib symptoms in check.

What Food to Eat

High-Fiber Foods

Eating foods rich in fiber is super important for your heart and managing AFib. These foods can help lower your cholesterol and keep your digestive system healthy. some examples of these high-fiber foods include;

- ➢ Chickpeas

- ➢ Lentils

- ➢ Split peas

- ➢ Oats

- ➢ Apples

- ➢ Pears

- ➢ Almonds

- ➢ Chia seeds

➢ Brussels sprouts

➢ Avocado

➢ Blackberries

➢ Kidney beans

When you add these fiber-rich foods to your meals every day can give you lots of health benefits, like better heart health, keeping your blood sugar levels steady, and helping you manage your weight. By making high-fiber foods a priority in your AFib diet, you're taking a proactive step toward managing your condition and keeping your overall health in check.

Lean Proteins

Including lean proteins in your diet is key for keeping your heart healthy, as they're low in unhealthy fats and cholesterol, but packed with important nutrients like iron, zinc, and B vitamins. Here are some great options for lean proteins:

➢ White-fleshed fish

➢ Skinless white meat poultry

➢ Beans, peas, lentils

➢ Plain Greek yogurt

- ➢ Lean beef

- ➢ Eggs

Antioxidant-Rich Foods

Foods that are packed with antioxidants are really good for your heart and can help prevent AFib. These antioxidants fight off harmful free radicals that can damage your cells and lead to chronic diseases, adding these antioxidant-rich foods to your AFib diet, you're not only enjoying tasty and nutrient-packed meals, but you're also giving your heart some extra love and lowering your risk of developing AFib. A diet full of antioxidants is a smart choice for anyone who wants to boost their overall health;

- Blueberries

- Spices and herbs

- Fruits and berries

- Vegetables

- Nuts

- Seeds

Foods to avoid for AFib

It's important for AFib patients to not only focus on eating heart-healthy foods but also to steer clear of certain foods that can worsen AFib symptoms or lead to heart issues. This means being mindful about avoiding sugary treats and drinks, processed foods, and beverages high in alcohol and caffeine.

Understanding what to stay away from and making smart choices about your diet, you're taking steps to better manage your AFib and improve your heart health. Finding the right balance in your diet that suits your needs is crucial for effectively managing your condition.

Sugary foods and drinks aren't great for your heart health and can increase the risk of AFib. They can lead to heart disease, weight gain, and other health problems and as such should be avoided;

- Puddings

- Milkshakes

- Ice cream

- Fruit juices

- Sugary sodas

- Candy

- Cakes

- Cookies

- Pies

- Sweet rolls

- Pastries

- Doughnuts

- Sweetened dairy desserts like ice cream and yogurt

- Sweetened drinks like sodas, sports drinks, energy drinks, and juice drinks

To cut down on sugar, you can:

- Avoid processed foods

- Check food labels for added sugars

- Limit sugary drinks

- Swap sugary snacks for healthier options

Also, you can try reducing your intake of sugary foods and drinks.

Processed Foods:

Processed foods often contain lots of salt, preservatives, and other additives that aren't great for your heart. Examples of processed foods to steer clear of include sugary drinks, deli meats, frozen meals, packaged snacks, and most breakfast cereals. Ultra-processed foods like chicken nuggets, hot dogs, and potato chips are also not the best choices.

Cutting back on processed foods and choosing fresh, whole foods instead, you're doing your heart a favor and lowering your risk of developing AFib. Pick foods that are packed with nutrients and are minimally processed to give your body what it needs to stay healthy and manage your AFib effectively.

Alcohol and Caffeine:

Alcohol and caffeine can be risky for people with AFib since they can trigger AFib episodes and make the condition worse. It's important to limit how much alcohol you drink and keep an eye on your caffeine intake, as both can worsen AFib symptoms and lead to heart problems. To reduce your risk of AFib episodes and manage your condition better, think about cutting back on alcohol or caffeine. By being mindful of these potential triggers, you're taking charge of your AFib and supporting your heart health.

Red Meat;

Red meats like beef or lamb usually have more saturated fat compared to white meat. Saturated fat can bump up your cholesterol levels, which can increase your risk of AFib. Choosing plant-based protein instead of red meat might help lower your cholesterol levels.

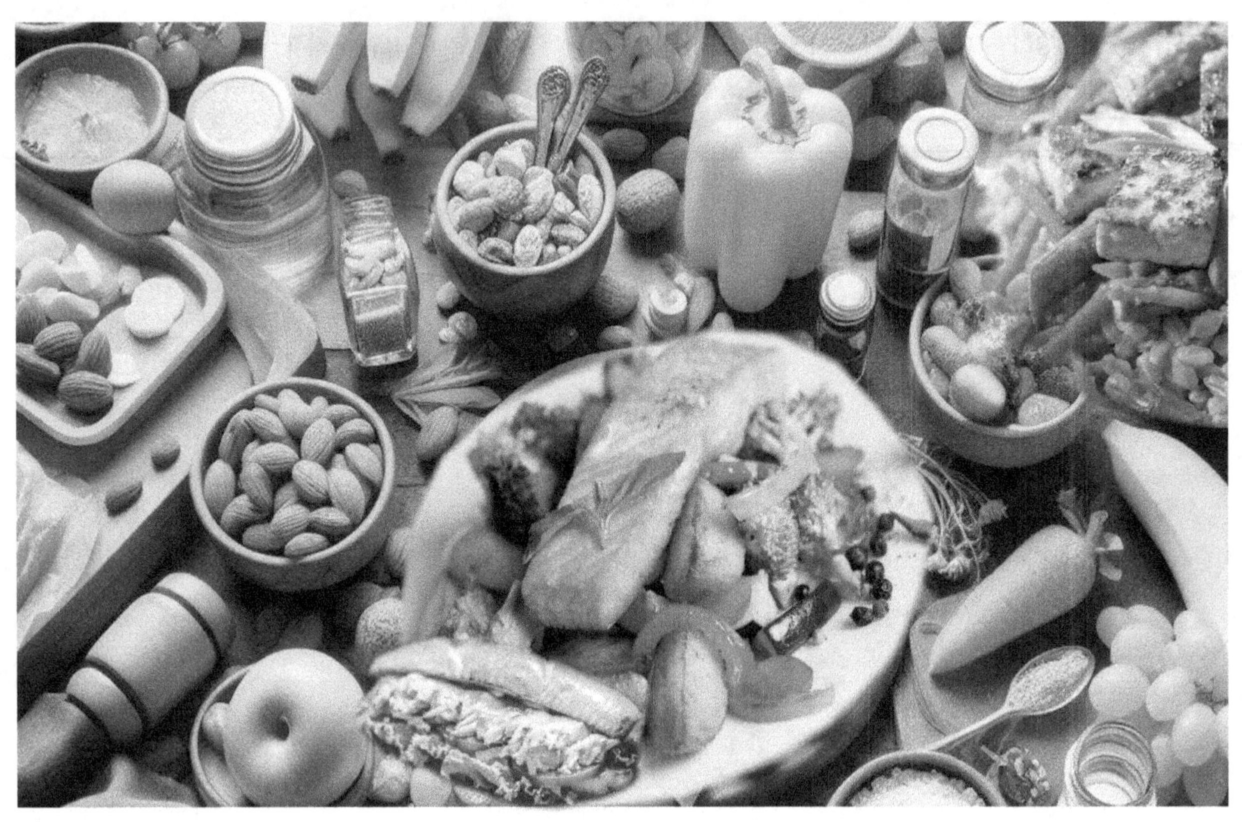

DIET AND RECIPES FOR AFIB

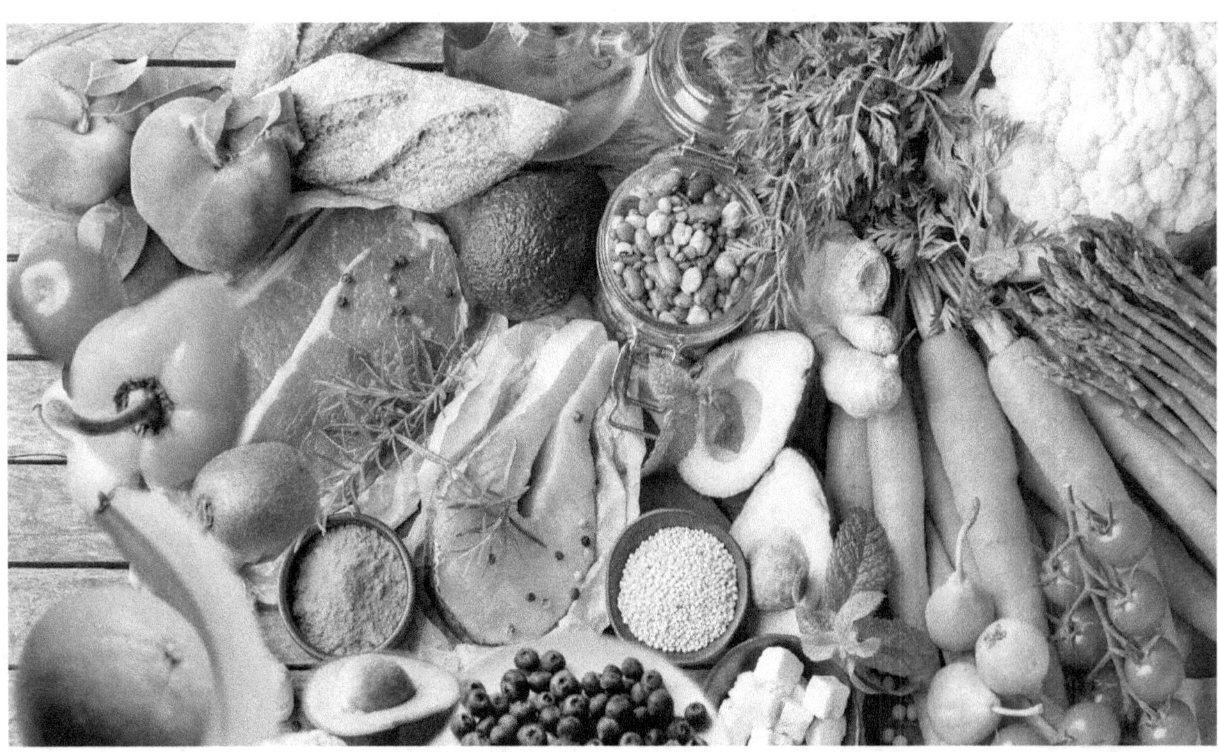

Losing weight isn't just about cutting calories or swapping out foods. It's a bit more complicated than that. Your weight can be influenced by things like how stressed you are, how well you sleep, how active you are, and even when you eat your meals. Studies have shown that eating more of your calories earlier in the day might lead to less weight gain compared to eating them later in the evening. Also, not all calories are the same when it comes to gaining weight. The mix of fats, proteins, and carbs you eat can affect your metabolism and how much weight you lose.

Most experts agree that processed foods and added sugars are big factors in the obesity problem we're facing today. Processing foods can strip away some of the good stuff they naturally have. For example, drinking apple juice gives you a big hit of sugar that can spike your insulin levels. But if you eat a whole, unprocessed apple instead, you get that same sugar along with fiber, which helps to even out the insulin spike. And sometimes, combining certain foods can lessen their negative effects. Like dipping bread in vinegar, which can help to lower the impact of the carbs in the bread on your metabolism.

These recipes are a collection of my dedicated years and experience in serving individuals both in the health sector and AFib persons.

Spicy Grilled Chicken with Black Bean Chilaquiles

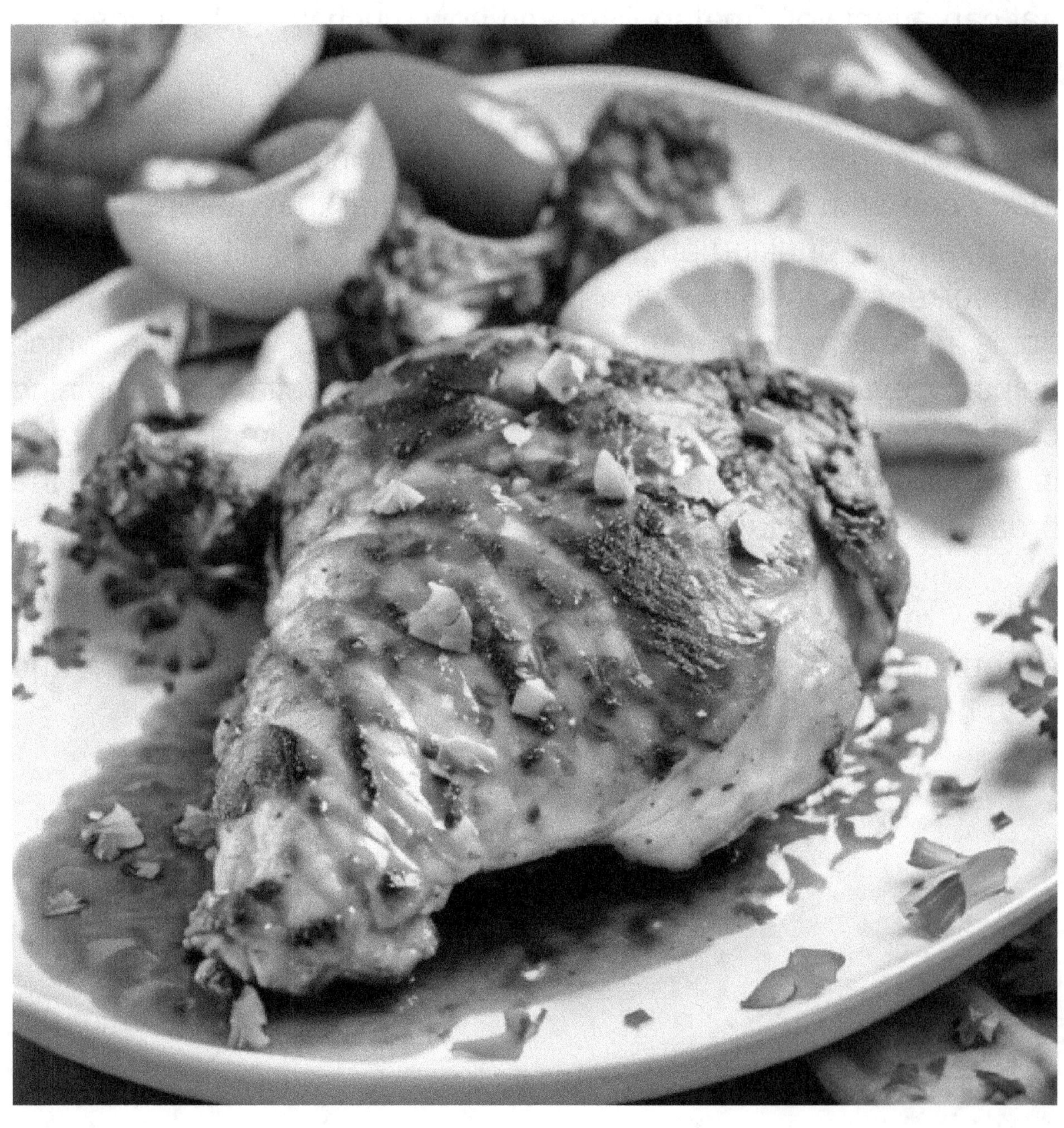

To make a healthy Spicy Grilled Chicken with Black Bean Chilaquiles, a very delicious and spicy grilled chicken dish that will leave your taste buds tingling follow these guidelines;

I. Instead of traditional fried tortillas, use whole grain or corn tortillas. Bake or air-fry them until crispy to reduce added fats.

II. Toppings: Opt for lighter toppings such as fresh salsa, diced tomatoes, onions, and cilantro, adding sliced avocado can provide healthy fats.

III. Seasonings: Use homemade spice blends or low-sodium seasoning mixes to control the sodium content. Minimize the use of salt and opt for fresh herbs and spices for flavor.

IV. Grilled Chicken: Marinate the chicken with herbs, spices, and a small amount of healthy oil instead of store-bought marinades high in sodium and sugar.

V. Beans: Choose low-sodium canned black beans or cook dried beans from scratch to control the sodium content. Rinse canned beans thoroughly before using them to remove excess salt.

VI. Vegetables: Increase the vegetable content by adding extra bell peppers, onions, spinach, or zucchini to the dish for added fiber and nutrients.

VII.   Portion Control: Pay attention to portion sizes to avoid overeating. Serve smaller portions of the chilaquiles and fill the rest of your plate with a variety of colorful vegetables.

Main Dish

Ingredients:

- 4 boneless, skinless chicken breasts

- 8 whole grain or corn tortillas

- 1 can (15 ounces) low-sodium black beans, drained and rinsed

- 1 red bell pepper, diced

- 1 yellow bell pepper, diced

- 1 onion, diced

- 2 cloves garlic, minced

- 1 jalapeño pepper, seeded and minced (optional for extra spice)

- 1 tablespoon olive oil

- 1 teaspoon chili powder

- 1 teaspoon ground cumin

- 1/2 teaspoon paprika

- Salt and pepper to taste

- Fresh cilantro, chopped, for garnish

- Lime wedges, for serving1/2 teaspoon black pepper

Preparation / direction

- Preheat your grill to medium-high heat. Season the chicken breasts with chili powder, cumin, paprika, salt, and pepper. Grill the chicken for 6-8 minutes per side, or until cooked through. Remove from the grill and let rest for a few minutes before slicing into strips.

- While the chicken is grilling, preheat your oven to 375°F (190°C). Cut the tortillas into wedges and spread them out on a baking sheet. Bake for 8-10 minutes, or until crispy and golden brown.

- In a large skillet, heat the olive oil over medium heat. Add the diced onion, bell peppers, garlic, and jalapeño (if using). Sauté for 5-6 minutes, or until the vegetables are softened.

- Add the black beans to the skillet and season with salt and pepper. Cook for an additional 2-3 minutes, until heated through.

- Once the tortilla chips are crispy, remove them from the oven and transfer them to a large mixing bowl. Add the cooked vegetables and black beans to the bowl and toss to combine.

- Arrange the sliced grilled chicken on top of the tortilla mixture. Place the skillet back on the stovetop over low heat and warm the chicken and tortilla mixture for 2-3 minutes.

- Serve the Spicy Grilled Chicken with Black Bean Chilaquiles garnished with fresh cilantro and lime wedges on the side.

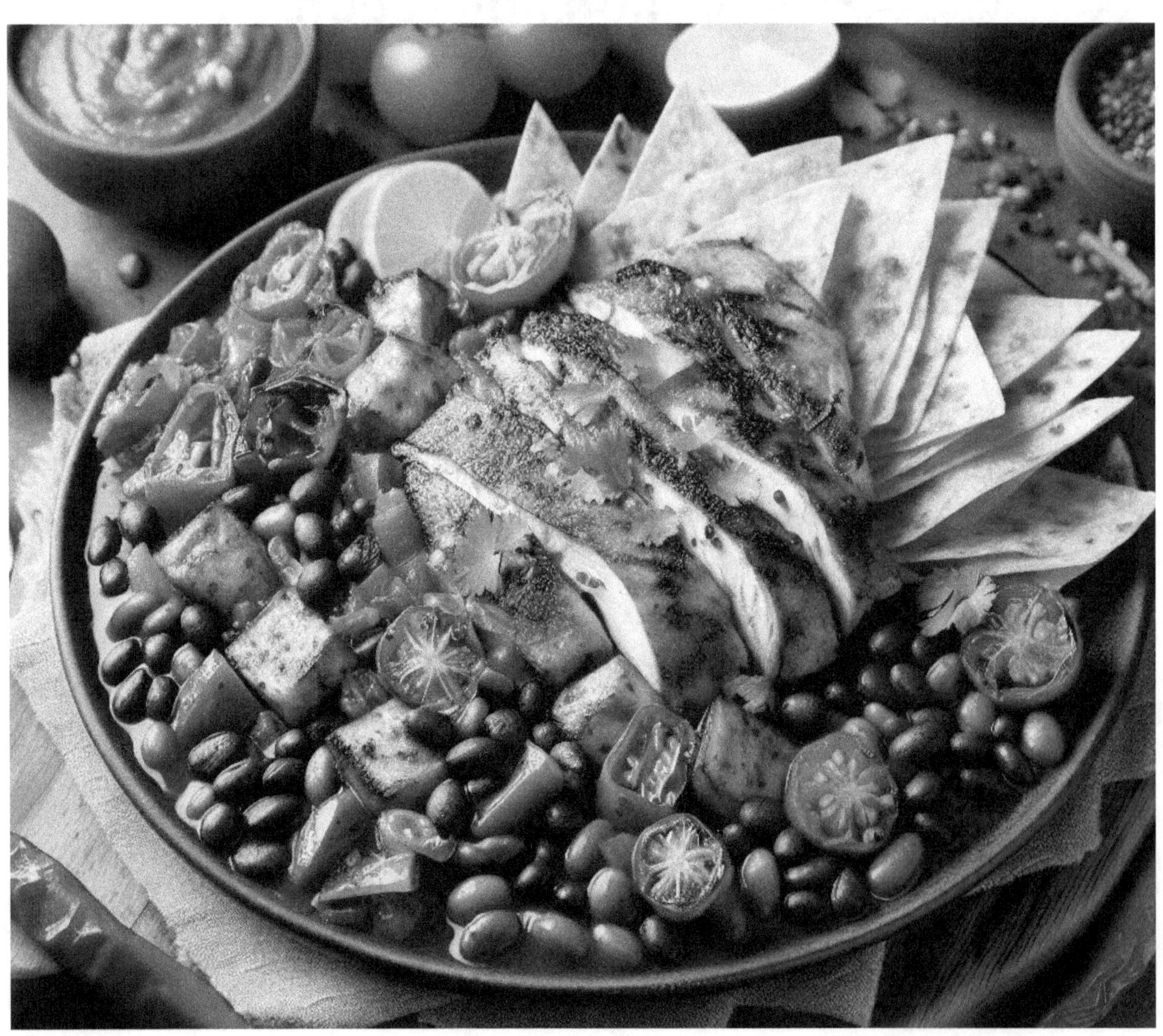

This is one of my favorite meals, because every recipe in it has a natural taste and like my doctor friend will always say "Lillian you are what you eat" so, let me tell you what you are eating in this meal;

Lean Protein: Grilled chicken breast is a lean source of protein, which is essential for muscle repair and maintenance. Protein helps keep you feeling full and satisfied, which can aid in weight management.

Whole Grains: Whole grain tortillas provide fiber, vitamins, and minerals that support heart health. Fiber helps regulate blood sugar levels and promotes digestive health, while whole grains have been linked to a reduced risk of heart disease.

Plant-Based Protein: Black beans are rich in plant-based protein, fiber, and antioxidants. They help lower cholesterol levels, regulate blood sugar, and support overall heart health.

Healthy Fats: Olive oil used for cooking adds heart-healthy monounsaturated fats to the dish. These fats help reduce inflammation and improve cholesterol levels.

Nutrient-Rich Vegetables: Bell peppers, onions, and jalapeños (if included) are packed with vitamins, minerals, and antioxidants. They contribute to overall health and may help reduce the risk of chronic diseases.

Low Sodium: By using low-sodium ingredients and minimizing added salt, this recipe helps control sodium intake, which is important for managing blood pressure and reducing the risk of stroke.

Balanced Meal: This recipe provides a balanced combination of protein, carbohydrates, and fats, along with plenty of vitamins and minerals from the vegetables. It can help stabilize blood sugar levels and promote overall well-being.

Nutritional Information

Calories	400-500 kcal
Protein	25-30 grams
Carbohydrates	40-50 grams
Fat	15-20 grams
Fiber	8-10 grams
Sodium	500-600 milligrams

Stir-fried ginger beef with grilled peppers

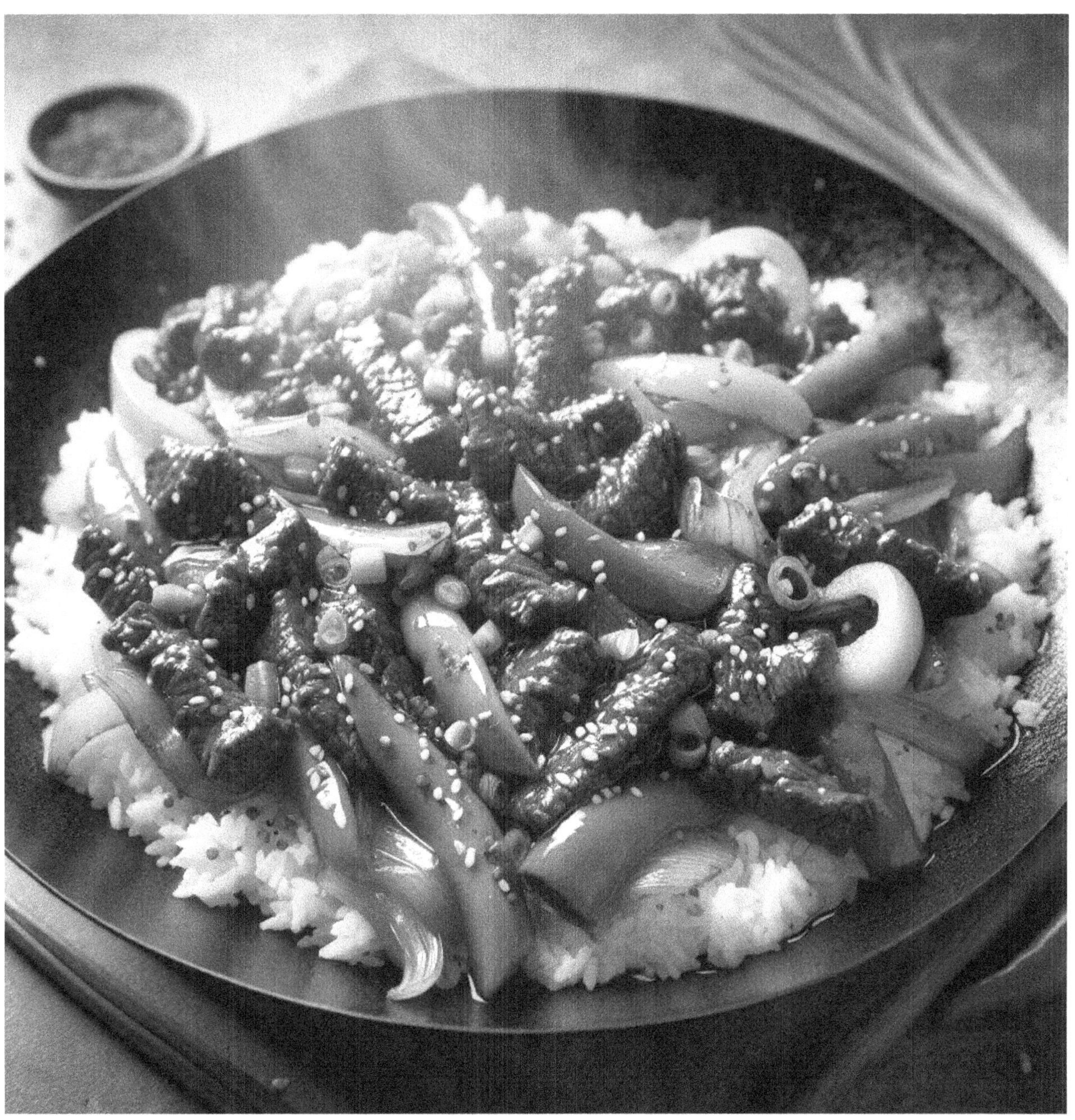

How you can make this meal depending on the ingredients and cooking methods is a great deal for a healthy heart. Ah, the stir-fried ginger beef with grilled peppers! It's a flavorful dish with a delightful combination of tender beef, zesty ginger, and smoky grilled peppers. While it may not be specifically aimed for those with AFib, it can still be enjoyed as part of a heart-healthy diet when prepared with lean beef and minimal added fats. Just be mindful of portion sizes and any additional sauces or seasonings to keep sodium levels in check.

Lean Beef: Choose lean cuts of beef, such as sirloin or tenderloin, and trim any visible fat to reduce saturated fat intake. Opting for lean protein sources can help lower cholesterol levels and support heart health.

Grilled Peppers: Grilled peppers add flavor and nutrition to the dish. Peppers are rich in vitamins A and C, as well as antioxidants, which can help reduce inflammation and protect against heart disease.

Ginger: Ginger is known for its anti-inflammatory properties and may help improve circulation and reduce the risk of blood clots. Including ginger in the stir-fry adds flavor without adding sodium or unhealthy fats.

Healthy Cooking Methods: Stir-frying with minimal oil and grilling the peppers can help reduce added fats and calories in the dish. Avoid excessive use of oils high in saturated fats, such as coconut oil or palm oil, and instead use heart-healthy oils like olive oil or avocado oil sparingly.

Whole Grains: Consider serving the stir-fry over brown rice or quinoa instead of white rice. Whole grains are higher in fiber and nutrients, which can help regulate blood sugar levels and promote heart health.

Ingredients:

- 1 lb lean beef (such as sirloin or flank steak), thinly sliced

- 2 bell peppers (any color), sliced into strips

- 2 tablespoons low-sodium soy sauce

- 1 tablespoon grated fresh ginger

- 2 cloves garlic, minced

- 1 tablespoon olive oil

- Salt and pepper to taste

- Optional: sliced green onions for garnish

Preparation / Direction

- In a bowl, combine the sliced beef, soy sauce, grated ginger, and minced garlic. Allow the beef to marinate for at least 30 minutes in the refrigerator.

- Preheat your grill to medium-high heat. Lightly coat the bell pepper strips with olive oil and season with salt and pepper.

- Grill the bell pepper strips until they are tender and slightly charred, about 5-7 minutes per side. Remove from the grill and set aside.

- Heat the olive oil in a large skillet or wok over medium-high heat. Add the marinated beef slices to the skillet and stir-fry until they are cooked through and lightly browned, about 3-4 minutes.

- Add the grilled bell pepper strips to the skillet with the beef and toss to combine. Cook for an additional 1-2 minutes to heat everything through.

- Serve the stir-fried ginger beef and grilled peppers hot, garnished with sliced green onions if desired. Enjoy this delicious and heart-healthy meal with a side of brown rice or quinoa for added fiber and nutrients.

Sizzling Healthy Prawn Fajitas with Avocado

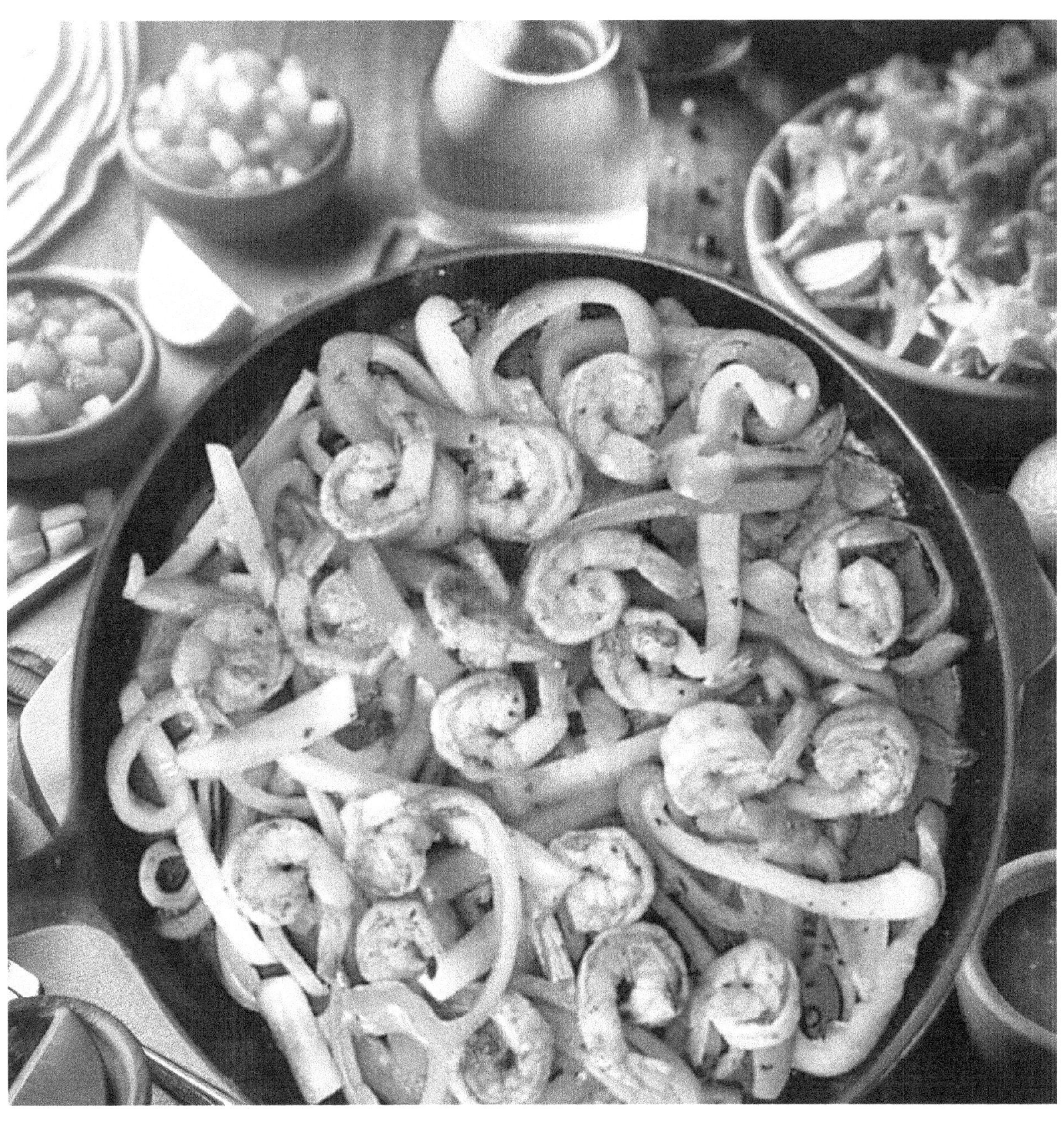

Sizzling Prawn Fajitas with avocado are great for AFib for several reasons. First and foremost, prawns are a lean source of protein, which is essential for muscle repair. Additionally, avocados are rich in heart-healthy fats, such as monounsaturated fats, which can help lower bad cholesterol levels and reduce the risk of heart disease, a common concern for individuals with AFib.

Ingredients:

- 1-pound large prawns, peeled and deveined

- 2 bell peppers (any color), sliced

- 1 onion, sliced

- 2 cloves garlic, minced

- 1 tablespoon olive oil

- 1 teaspoon ground cumin

- 1 teaspoon chili powder

- 1/2 teaspoon smoked paprika

- Salt and pepper to taste

- Whole wheat or whole grain tortillas

- Optional toppings: sliced avocado, salsa, Greek yogurt or low-fat sour cream, chopped cilantro

Direction / Preparation

- Heat olive oil in a large skillet over medium heat. Add minced garlic and cook for 1 minute until fragrant.

- Add sliced bell peppers and onions to the skillet. Cook for 5-7 minutes, stirring occasionally, until vegetables are tender-crisp.

- Push the vegetables to one side of the skillet and add prawns to the empty side. Season prawns with ground cumin, chili powder, smoked paprika, salt, and pepper. Cook for 2-3 minutes on each side until prawns are pink and opaque.

- Once prawns are cooked through, mix them with the vegetables in the skillet. Stir well to combine and heat through for another minute.

- Warm the whole wheat tortillas according to package instructions.

- Serve the sizzling prawn and vegetable mixture on warm tortillas. Top with optional toppings such as sliced avocado, salsa, Greek yogurt or low-fat sour cream, and chopped cilantro.

- Roll up the tortillas and enjoy your heart-healthy Sizzling Prawn Fajitas

This recipe provides a balance of lean protein from prawns, fiber and nutrients from vegetables, and whole grains from whole wheat tortillas. Let's look at some of the important nutrients in this dish.

I. **prawns** are a great source of lean protein, which is important for maintaining muscle health and our energy levels. Plus, they're low in saturated fat, which is beneficial for heart health.

II. **Avocado**, a key ingredient in this dish, is packed with heart-healthy monounsaturated fats, which help to lower bad cholesterol levels and reduce the risk of heart disease, also avocados are rich in potassium, a mineral that plays a crucial role in regulating blood pressure.

III. **The colorful bell peppers and onions** used in fajitas are not only flavorful but also provide essential vitamins and antioxidants, supporting general health and immune function.

IV.   **Serving** the fajitas with whole wheat tortillas adds fiber to the meal, promoting digestive health and helping to maintain stable blood sugar levels.

Talking about AFib, it's important to eat foods that are packed with nutrients. These are the foods that give you the most vitamins and minerals. Things like processed cereals, cookies, and candies don't have many nutrients. But foods like vegetables, fruits, nuts, seeds, lentils, and protein foods do.

When you eat more of these nutritious foods, your body gets a big boost of vitamins and minerals. This helps your body heal and get better. For AFib, some of the best nutrients are vitamin C, silica, potassium, calcium, and magnesium. So, it's good to eat foods that have these nutrients, for examples;

- Cantaloupe

- Watermelon

- Pears

- Dairy Products

- Dandelion Greens

- Cucumbers

- Blueberries

- Raspberries

- Grapefruit

- Limes

➢ Parsnips

➢ Celery

➢ Honeydew Melon

➢ Peaches

➢ Spinach

➢ Kale

➢ Almonds

➢ Strawberries

➢ Blackberries

➢ Oranges

➢ Lemons

➢ Bell Peppers

➢ Carrots

These are all yummy foods that can help you feel better. Do you think you could try eating some of these every day? If you do, you might notice a big improvement in your health

Honey Fruit Salad

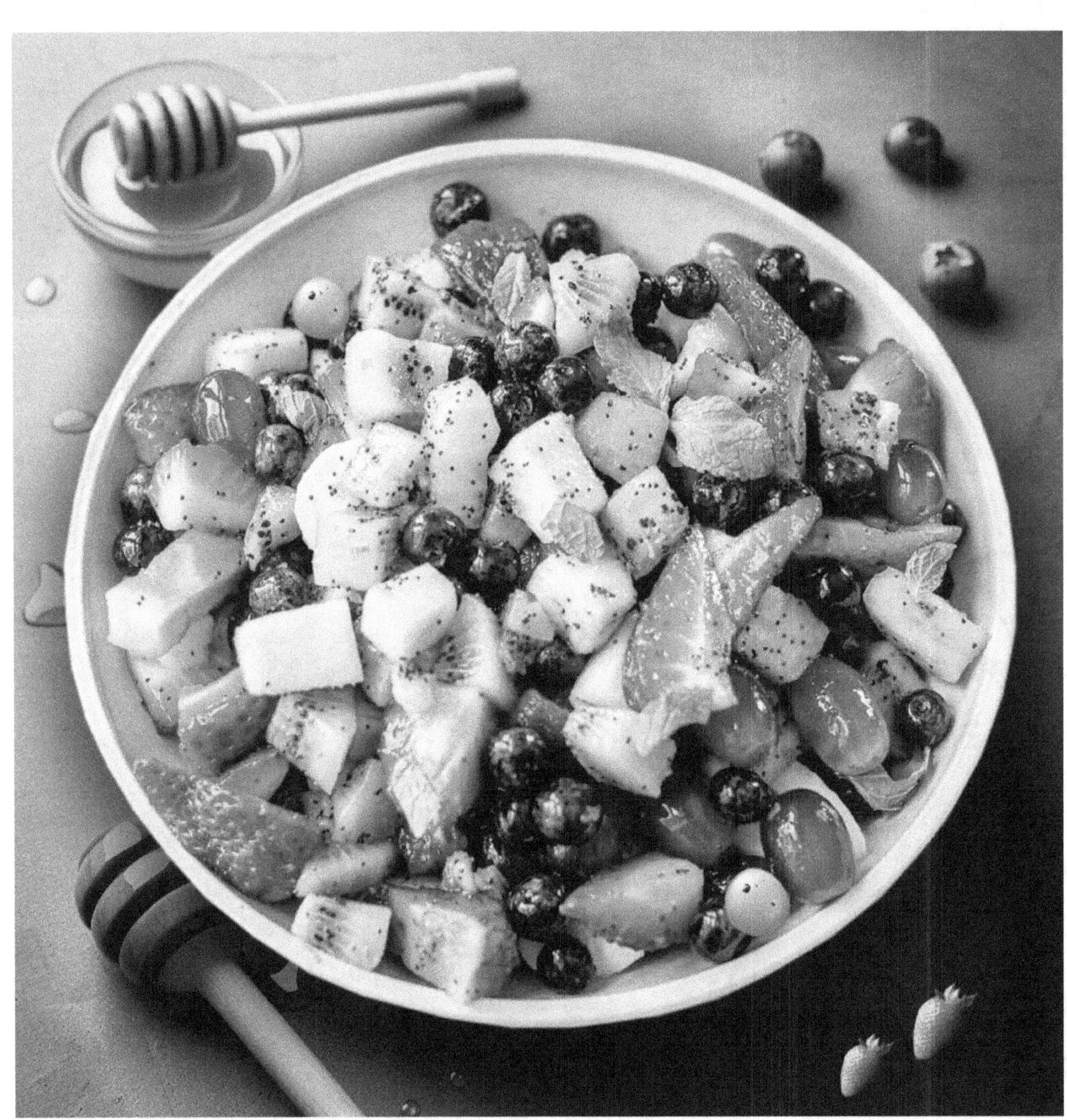

This simple yet delightful fruit salad brings together a medley of fresh flavors, including watermelon, blueberries, cantaloupe, kiwi, pineapple chunks, mandarin oranges, and grapes, all tossed in a refreshing lime and honey dressing.

Heading out to pick berries is a classic summer pastime, but what do you do when you return home with bags full of berries just waiting to be used? If you're anything like me, you find yourself munching on them by the handful while hurriedly searching Pinterest for fresh recipes to try before those berries start to lose their luster. Time flies when you're having berry fun, doesn't it?

This fruit salad is ideal for those moments when you find yourself overwhelmed with an abundance of fruit and are unsure what to do with it. It also serves as a wonderfully effortless side dish for cookouts, backyard BBQs, picnics, or gatherings. When preparing a fruit salad, it's essential to use fresh, seasonal fruit to achieve the tastiest outcome.

Ingredients:

- 2 cups of mixed berries (such as strawberries, blueberries, raspberries, and blackberries)

- 1 cup of diced watermelon

- 1 cup of diced cantaloupe

- 1 cup of diced pineapple

* 1 cup of diced kiwi

* 1 cup of grapes, halved

* 1 tablespoon of honey (optional)

* Juice of 1 lime

* Natural honey

Preparation / Direction

* Wash all the fruits thoroughly.

* Prepare the fruits by slicing and dicing them into bite-sized pieces.

* In a large mixing bowl, combine all the fruits.

* Squeeze the lime juice over the fruits to add a refreshing citrus flavor. You can also drizzle honey over the fruits if you prefer a sweeter taste, but this is optional.

* Gently toss the fruits until they are well combined.

* Serve the fruit salad immediately or chill it in the refrigerator for about 30 minutes before serving for a refreshing treat.

Feel free to regard all the fruits in this recipe as my suggestions! While I personally adore this particular combination and find it perfectly delightful, feel empowered to swap out any fruits you prefer or have readily available in your fridge, provided it one of the fruits I listed earlier. So why do I particularly adore these salads? And what benefits does it holds in our health?

1) **Natural Sweetness:** Honey adds a touch of sweetness to the fruit salad without the need for refined sugars. Unlike processed sugars, honey contains antioxidants and other beneficial compounds that may support heart health when consumed in moderation.

2) **Nutrient-Rich Fruits:** The salad features a variety of fruits rich in vitamins, minerals, and antioxidants essential for cardiovascular health. Fruits like berries, kiwi, oranges, and grapes provide potassium, vitamin C, fiber, and other nutrients beneficial for managing AFib and promoting our heart health.

3) **Hydration:** Fruits like watermelon, oranges, and grapes have high water content, aiding in hydration. Proper hydration is crucial for maintaining healthy blood pressure levels and supporting cardiovascular function, which is especially important for individuals with AFib.

4) **Anti-Inflammatory Properties:** Honey contains antioxidants and anti-inflammatory compounds that may help reduce inflammation in the body. Chronic inflammation is linked to various cardiovascular conditions, including AFib. Consuming honey in moderation as part of a heart-healthy

diet may help mitigate inflammation and support heart health.

5) **Digestive Health:** Honey has been traditionally used to support digestive health and may help soothe the digestive tract. Incorporating honey into the fruit salad can provide gentle support for digestive function and well-being.

Nutritional Information	
Calories	100-150 kcal
Protein	1-2 grams
Carbohydrates	25-30 grams
Fat	0-1 grams
Fiber	2-4 grams
Sodium	0-5 milligrams

Raitha with cucumber

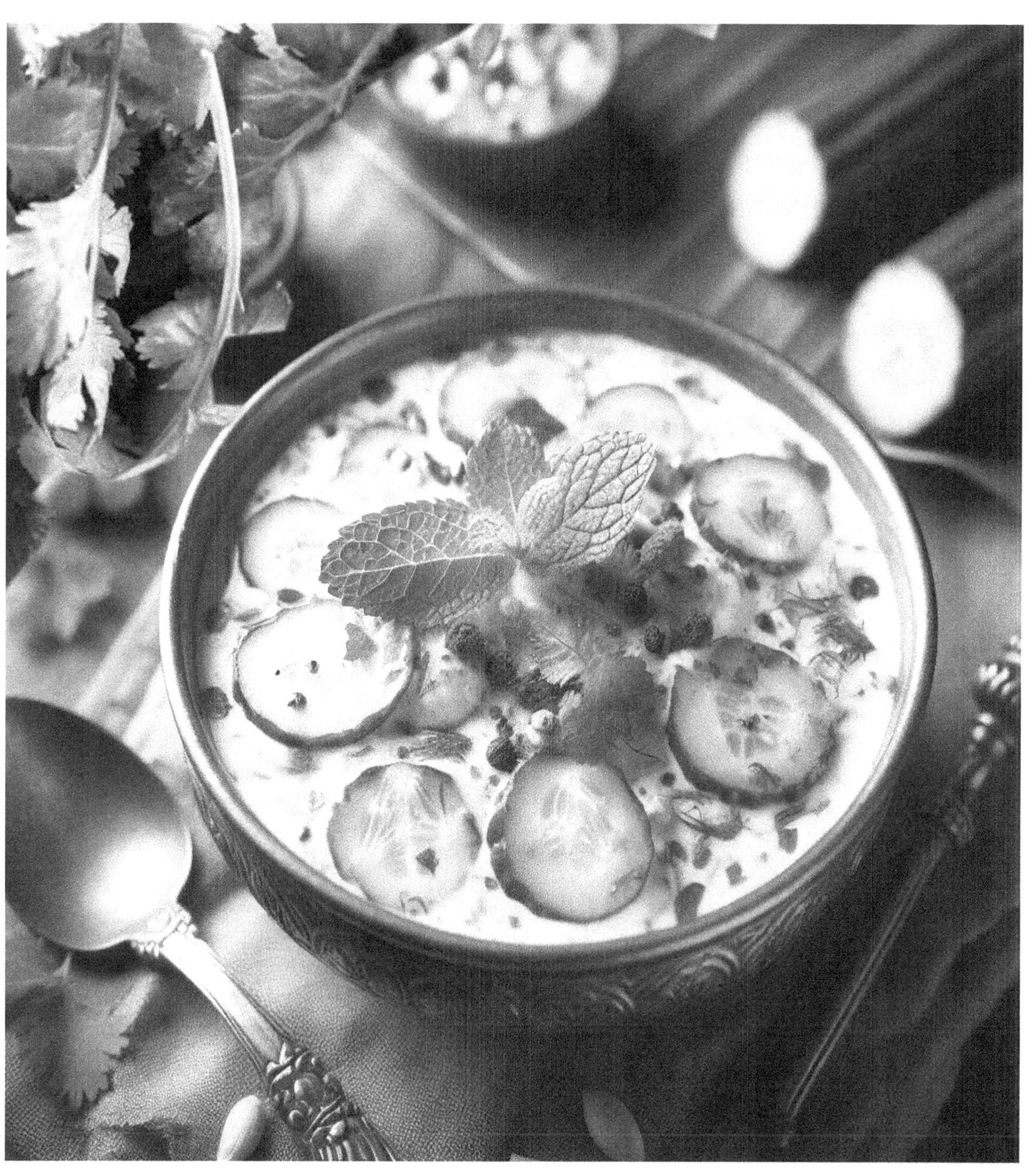

This refreshing cucumber raita is the perfect complement to spicy Indian cuisine. Featuring finely grated crisp cucumbers mixed with creamy plain yogurt, and seasoned with a touch of garlic and cumin, this recipe is a delightful addition to any meal.

Prepare this cucumber raita recipe ahead of time to allow the flavors to meld and develop in the fridge. Feel free to adjust the amount of fresh mint according to your preference, as dried mint doesn't offer the same flavor profile.

Raita, a gluten-free side dish made from yogurt, is commonly served alongside Indian meals and shares similarities with Tzatziki, a Greek yogurt side dish. This cooling accompaniment pairs well with spicy Indian dishes like curries, vegetables, dals, and biryanis. Typically comprising yogurt, vegetables or fruit, and herbs, raita recipes are quick to assemble and require no cooking, taking less than ten minutes to prepare. In my household, cucumber raita reigns supreme due to its simplicity, no-cook nature, and universal appeal.

Ingredients:

- 1 cup plain yogurt (preferably low-fat or non-fat)

- 1 cucumber, grated or finely chopped
- 1 tablespoon chopped fresh cilantro (coriander)

- 1/2 teaspoon roasted cumin powder

- 1/2 teaspoon salt, or to taste

- 1/4 teaspoon black pepper

- A pinch of cayenne pepper (optional)

- 1 tablespoon finely chopped mint leaves (optional)

- 1/2 teaspoon chaat masala (optional, for extra flavor)

Preparation / Directions

- In a mixing bowl, whisk the yogurt until smooth.

- Add the grated or chopped cucumber to the yogurt and mix well.

- Stir in the chopped cilantro, roasted cumin powder, salt, black pepper, and any optional ingredients like mint leaves or chaat masala.

- Adjust the seasoning according to your taste preferences.
- Refrigerate the raita for at least 30 minutes to allow the flavors to meld together.

- Serve chilled as a refreshing side dish with meals, particularly spicy or flavorful dishes.

Advance preparation: keep for a few days in the refrigerator but will become a little watery. Stir well before serving. An Indian chef of mine would say "I understand that the quintessential raita flavor comes from the tempering process known as 'vagurney'. This involves frying mustard seeds and cumin seeds in oil for about 45 seconds, adding the mustard seeds 15 seconds before the cumin for optimal flavor infusion".

This Cucumber Raita recipe is an excellent meal not just for individuals with AFib but the family as well, so what does this recipe helps us with in our body and health;

Low in Sodium: The recipe uses minimal salt, which is beneficial for those with AFib, as excessive sodium intake can contribute to high blood pressure, a risk factor for AFib.

High in Potassium: Cucumbers are naturally rich in potassium, a mineral that helps regulate heart rhythm and can counteract the effects of sodium on blood pressure. Maintaining a good balance of potassium and sodium is important for heart health, especially for those with AFib.

Cooling and Hydrating: Cucumbers have a high-water content, making this raita a hydrating dish that can help prevent dehydration, a potential trigger for AFib episodes. Additionally, the cooling properties of cucumber can provide relief from inflammation or discomfort associated with AFib.

Digestive Aid: Yogurt, the main ingredient in raita, contains probiotics that support gut health and digestion. Digestive issues can sometimes exacerbate AFib symptoms, so consuming probiotic-rich foods like yogurt can be beneficial.

Versatile and Flavorful: This raita recipe is versatile and can be customized with additional herbs and spices according to taste preferences. It can complement a variety of dishes, including spicy or flavorful meals, without adding excessive calories or unhealthy fats.

Nutritional Information

Calories	50-80 kcal
Protein	2-4 grams
Carbohydrates	3-5 grams
Fat	3-5 grams
Fiber	1-2 grams
Sodium:	20-50 milligrams

Red Plum Compote with Brown Rice

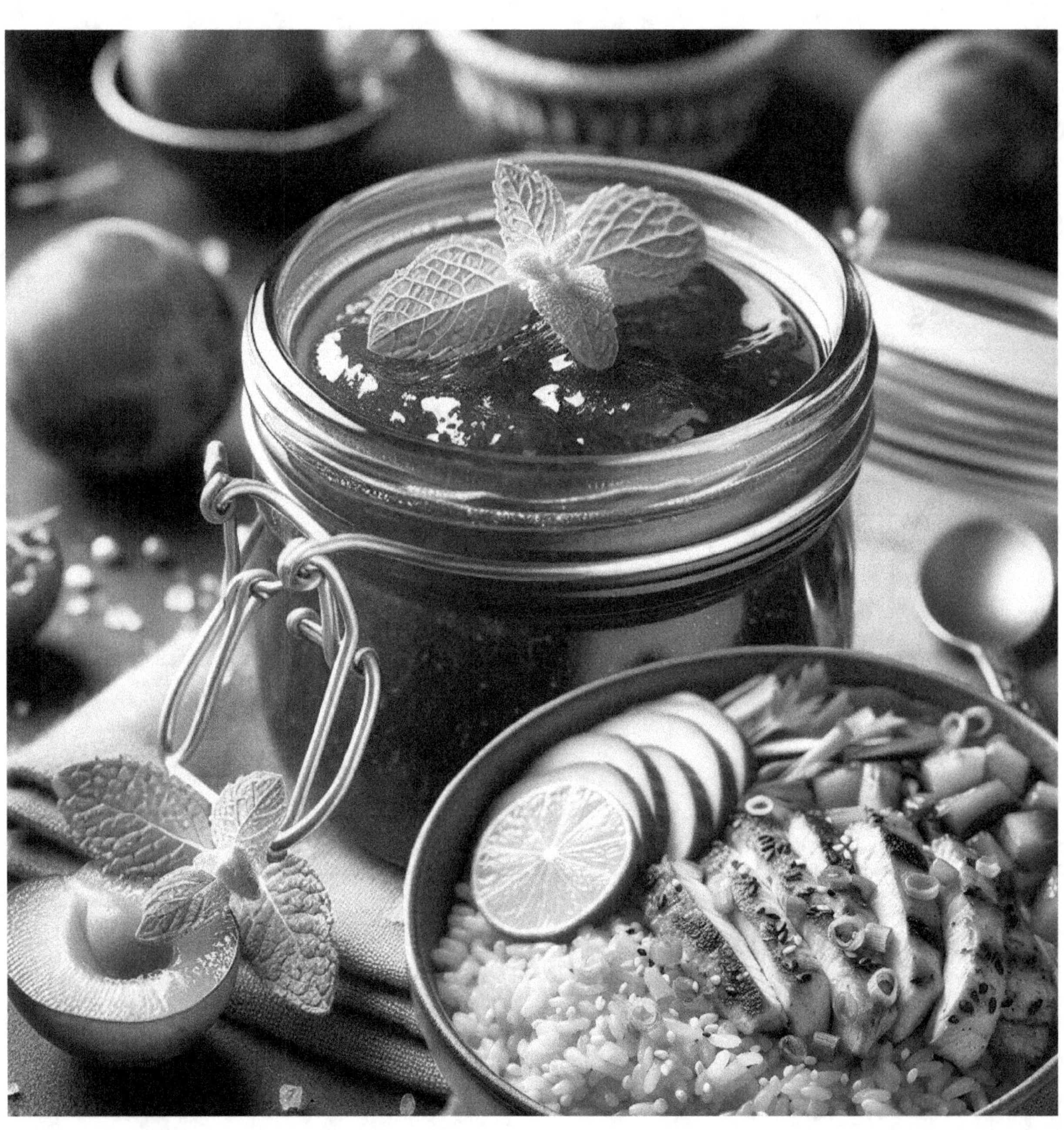

To create a red plum compote with brown rice friendlier, start by cutting back on added sugar or opting for natural sweeteners like honey or maple syrup in moderation. Spice things up by adding cinnamon or ginger, not only for flavor but also for potential heart health benefits. Boost the nutritional profile by tossing in other heart-healthy fruits such as berries or apples, which bring fiber and antioxidants to the table. And remember, watch your portions to avoid overdoing it on the sugar. With these tweaks, whip up a red plum compote that's both tasty and kind to your heart

This recipe focuses on reducing added sugars and incorporating natural sweeteners. These adjustments help lower the overall sugar content, which is beneficial for managing AFib. Additionally, the inclusion of spices like cinnamon or ginger not only enhances the flavor but also offers potential health benefits for heart health. moreover, adding heart-healthy fruits such as berries or apples increases the fiber and antioxidant content of the compote. By being mindful of portion sizes and making these adjustments, this red plum compote becomes a delicious and supportive option.

Ingredients:

- 6-8 ripe red plums, pitted and sliced

- 2-3 tablespoons honey or maple syrup (adjust to taste)

- 1 teaspoon ground cinnamon

- 1/2 teaspoon ground ginger

- 1/4 cup water

- Optional: Fresh berries or diced apples for added fiber and antioxidants

Preparation / Direction

- In a saucepan, combine the sliced red plums, honey or maple syrup, ground cinnamon, ground ginger, and water.

- Stir the mixture gently to coat the plums evenly with the sweetener and spices.

- Place the saucepan over medium heat and bring the mixture to a gentle simmer.

- Reduce the heat to low and let the compote simmer uncovered for about 15-20 minutes, stirring occasionally, until the plums have softened and the mixture has thickened slightly.

- Taste the compote and adjust the sweetness or spice levels if needed by adding more honey, cinnamon, or ginger.

- If desired, stir in some fresh berries or diced apples for added texture, fiber, and antioxidants.

- Remove the compote from the heat and let it cool slightly before serving.

- Serve the red plum compote warm or chilled as a topping for yogurt, oatmeal, pancakes, or desserts.

Benefits of this Recipe

Reduced Added Sugar: By using natural sweeteners like honey or maple syrup and reducing the amount of added sugar, this compote helps to lower overall sugar intake. Excessive sugar consumption can contribute to inflammation and negatively affect heart health, so reducing added sugars is beneficial for managing AFib.

Incorporation of Heart-Healthy Spices: The addition of ground cinnamon and ginger not only enhances the flavor of the compote but also provides potential health benefits. Cinnamon is known for its antioxidant properties and may help lower blood sugar levels and reduce inflammation, while ginger has anti-inflammatory and digestive benefits, which can support overall heart health.

Fiber and Antioxidants: Optionally adding fresh berries or diced apples to the compote increases its fiber content and antioxidant levels. Fiber is essential for digestive health and can help regulate blood sugar and cholesterol levels, while antioxidants help to reduce inflammation and protect against oxidative stress, both of which are important for managing AFib

Home-made Vegetable Pizza

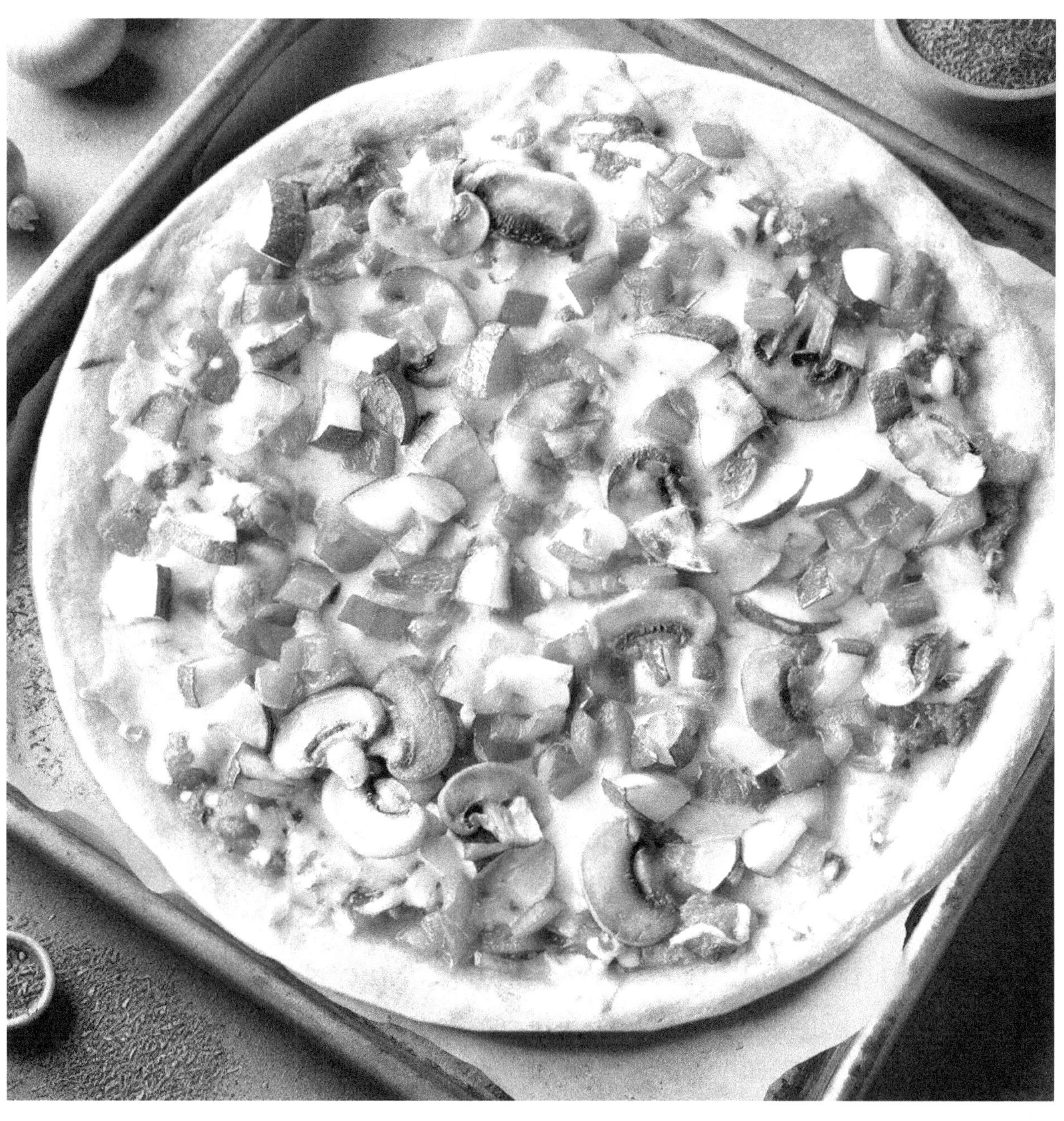

Creating a pizza might appear straightforward, but for individuals managing atrial fibrillation (AFib), every ingredient holds significant importance. Initially, the crust plays a pivotal role. Opting for whole grain or whole wheat crust introduces a wealth of nutrients like fiber, which promotes digestion and heart health.

Throughout my culinary journey, I've encountered numerous veggie pizzas. However, truly exceptional ones are somewhat scarce. In this homemade veggie pizza recipe, I've amalgamated all my favorite ingredients from years of experience to craft the ultimate homemade veggie pizza. It's a recipe I deem remarkable, achievable for anyone to whip up at home swiftly and effortlessly.

This homemade veggie pizza recipe promises delight for all, appealing to both vegetarians and non-vegetarians alike. Bursting with freshness and an array of flavors, it features artichokes, olives, red onions, spinach, and cherry tomatoes. Additionally, it boasts a delectable tomato sauce base complemented by creamy mozzarella cheese. These vegetables are brimming with antioxidants, vitamins, and minerals that combat inflammation and promote cardiovascular health.

When considering protein options, opt for lean choices like grilled chicken breast, turkey sausage, or tofu. These sources provide essential nutrients without the unhealthy fats typically found in red meats, aiding in the maintenance of optimal cholesterol levels.

Moving on to the sauce, traditional tomato sauce suffices, but homemade versions with reduced sugar and salt content are preferable. Alternatively, experiment with alternatives such as olive oil, pesto, or hummus, all of which boast lower sodium and sugar levels, thereby minimizing the exacerbation of AFib symptoms.

- 1 whole grain or whole wheat pizza crust

- 1 cup homemade or low-sugar tomato sauce

- 1 cup chopped mixed vegetables (such as bell peppers, mushrooms, onions, spinach, and cherry tomatoes)

- 1/2 cup shredded low-fat mozzarella cheese

- 1 tablespoon olive oil

- 1 teaspoon garlic powder

- 1 teaspoon dried basil

- Salt and pepper to taste

- Fresh basil leaves for garnish (optional)

Preparation / Direction

- Preheat the oven: Preheat your oven to the temperature specified on the pizza crust packaging.
- Prepare the crust: Place the whole grain pizza crust on a baking sheet or pizza stone. If using a pre-made crust, follow the instructions for pre-baking, if necessary.

- Spread the sauce: Evenly spread the homemade or low-sugar tomato sauce over the surface of the pizza crust, leaving a small border around the edges.

- Add the vegetables: Sprinkle the chopped mixed vegetables over the sauce, distributing them evenly across the pizza. Get creative with your vegetable toppings and use a variety of colors for added nutrition.

- Top with cheese: Sprinkle the shredded low-fat mozzarella cheese over the vegetables, covering the entire pizza evenly.

- Season and drizzle: Drizzle the olive oil over the top of the pizza, then sprinkle with garlic powder, dried basil, salt, and pepper to taste.

- Bake the pizza: Place the pizza in the preheated oven and bake according to the instructions on the pizza crust packaging, typically around 12-15 minutes, or until the crust is golden brown and the cheese is bubbly and melted.

- Garnish and serve: Remove the pizza from the oven and let it cool slightly. Garnish with fresh basil leaves, if desired, then slice and serve hot.

Jeweled Giant Couscous with Grilled Chicken Skewers

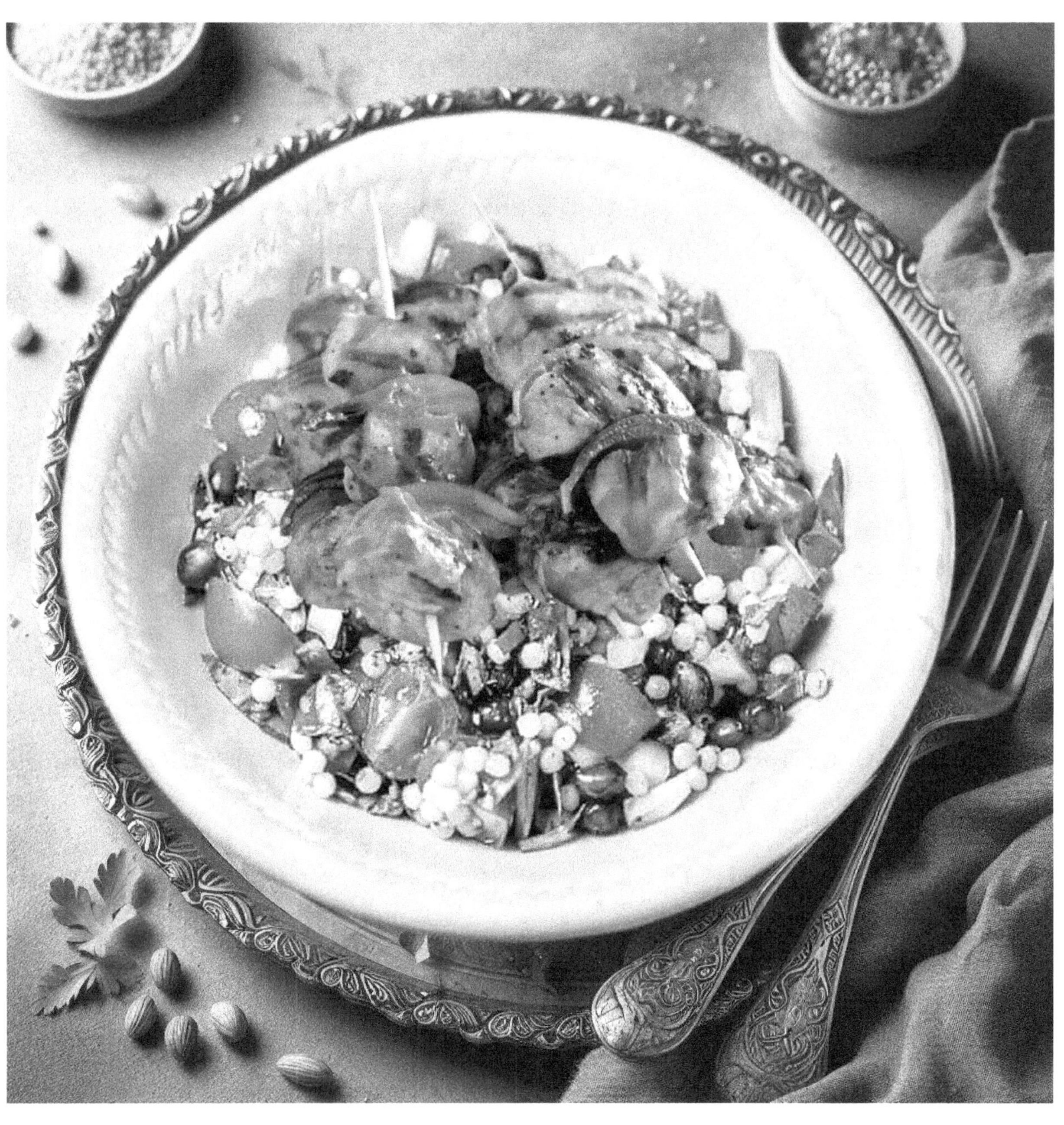

I did say Yes to jeweled giant couscous with grilled chicken skewers anytime, any day! depending on the ingredients and how I prepare it. Here's why it can be a suitable choice for you;

Whole Grain Couscous: Giant couscous, similar to regular couscous, is often made from whole wheat or whole grain semolina, providing fiber and complex carbohydrates that support heart health.

Grilled Chicken: Lean proteins like grilled chicken are essential for a heart-healthy diet. Chicken is low in saturated fats and provides essential nutrients like protein, which helps with muscle repair and satiety.

Vegetables and Fruits: If the dish includes vegetables and fruits, such as colorful bell peppers, cherry tomatoes, or pomegranate seeds, it adds essential vitamins, minerals, and antioxidants that support overall health and may help manage AFib.

Nuts and Seeds: Some recipes include nuts or seeds like almonds or pine nuts, which provide healthy fats, protein, and fiber. These can contribute to heart health when consumed in moderation.

Ingredients:

For Grilled Chicken Skewers:

- 2 boneless, skinless chicken breasts, cut into chunks

- 1 tablespoon olive oil

- 1 teaspoon paprika

- 1 teaspoon garlic powder

- 1 teaspoon ground cumin

- Salt and pepper to taste

- Wooden skewers, soaked in water for 30 minutes

For Jeweled Giant Couscous:

- 1 cup giant couscous

- 1 ½ cups water or low-sodium chicken broth

- 1 tablespoon olive oil

- 1 small red onion, finely chopped

- 1 garlic clove, minced

- 1/4 cup dried cranberries

- 1/4 cup chopped pistachios

- 1/4 cup pomegranate seeds

- Juice of 1 lemon

- Salt and pepper to taste

- Fresh parsley or mint leaves for garnish (optional)

Preparation / Direction

- Marinate the Chicken: In a bowl, combine olive oil, paprika, garlic powder, cumin, salt, and pepper. Add the chicken chunks and toss to coat. Cover and refrigerate for at least 30 minutes, or overnight for best flavor.

- Prepare the Giant Couscous: In a saucepan, bring water or chicken broth to a boil. Add the giant couscous and reduce heat to low. Simmer, covered, for 8-10 minutes or until the couscous is tender and has absorbed the liquid. Remove from heat and let it sit, covered, for 5 minutes. Fluff the couscous with a fork.

- Grill the Chicken: Preheat grill or grill pan over medium-high heat. Thread the marinated chicken onto the soaked wooden skewers. Grill for 4-5 minutes on each side, or until cooked through and nicely charred. Remove from heat and set aside.

- Prepare the Couscous Salad: In a large skillet, heat olive oil over medium heat. Add chopped onion and garlic, and sauté until softened, about 3-4 minutes. Add the cooked giant couscous to the skillet along with dried cranberries, chopped pistachios, and pomegranate seeds. Cook for another 2-3 minutes, stirring occasionally.

- Assemble the Dish: Transfer the jeweled giant couscous to a serving platter. Arrange the grilled chicken skewers on top. Drizzle lemon juice over the couscous and chicken. Season with salt and pepper to taste.

- Garnish and Serve: Garnish with fresh parsley or mint leaves, if desired. Serve the Jeweled Giant Couscous with Grilled Chicken Skewers warm or at room temperature

Nutritional Information	
Calories	300-400 kcal per serving
Protein	20-25 grams
Carbohydrates	30-40 grams
Fat	10-15 grams
Fiber	3-5 grams
Sodium	300-500 milligrams

Mushroom & Tofu Stir-Fry

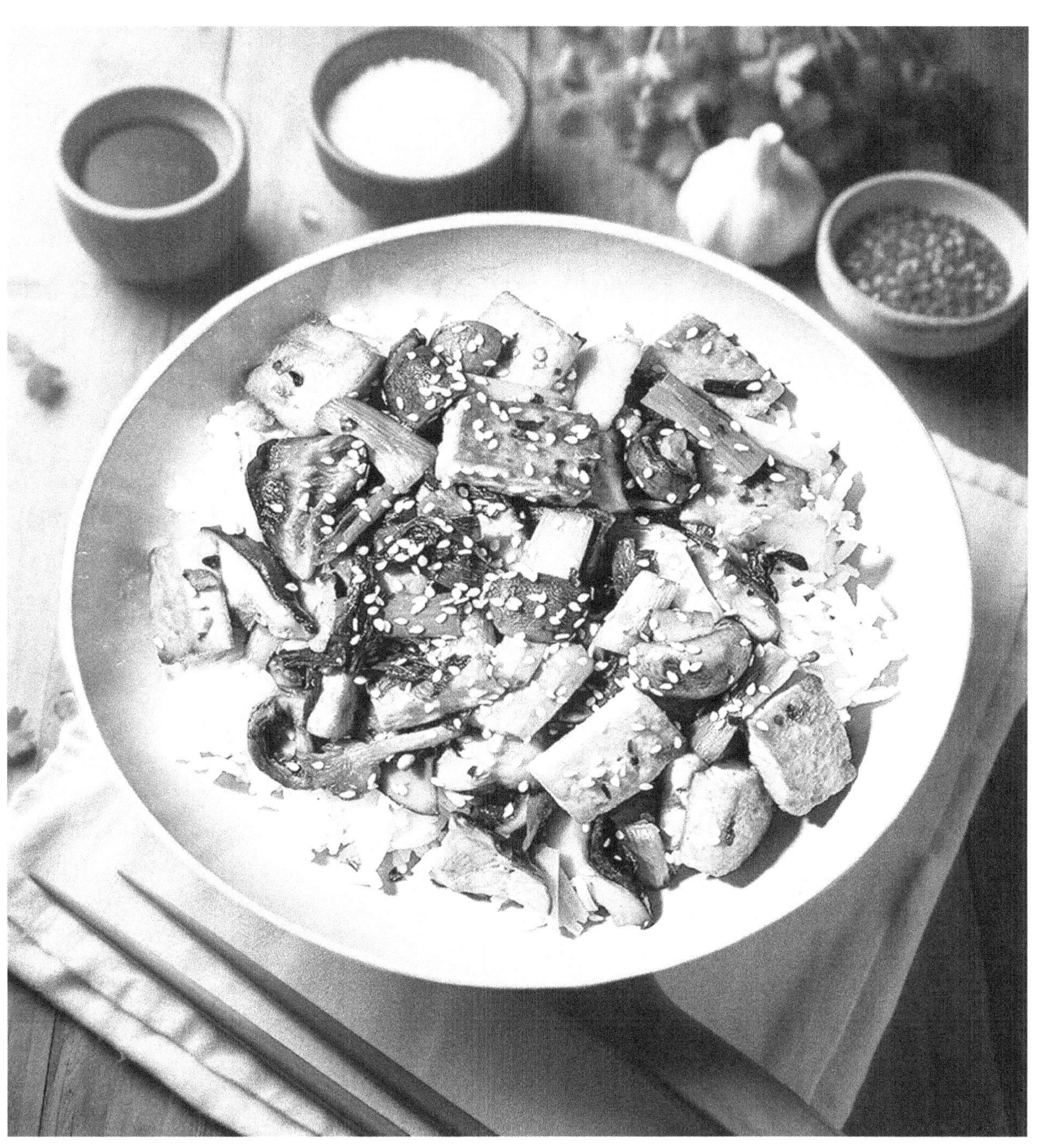

If you find yourself with some additional time prior to preparing this stir-fry, take the entire tofu block and place it between two layers of paper towels. Apply weight with a couple of large cans for 15 minutes. This step aids in removing excess water, enhancing the tofu's crispiness during the cooking process.

When recommending this dish, I'd emphasize its heart-healthy components, like tofu, which is a great plant-based source of protein, and mushrooms, which are loaded with vitamins and minerals. To make it even more suitable for someone with AFib, I will suggest using low-sodium soy sauce or tamari to control salt intake. Plus, adding plenty of colorful vegetables not only boosts the dish's nutritional value but also adds flavor and texture without relying on excess salt or unhealthy fats.

Cooking methods matter too. Stir-frying with minimal oil or using cooking spray can help keep added fats in check, and grilling or baking the tofu and mushrooms adds a delicious charred flavor without the need for frying.

Ultimately, it's all about balance and moderation. Enjoying this stir-fry as part of a well-rounded diet, along with plenty of other fruits, vegetables, whole grains, and lean proteins, can contribute to better heart health, why is why I will want you to pay a closed attention to the recipes.

Ingredients:

- 1 block (14 oz) firm tofu, pressed and cubed
- 8 oz mushrooms (such as button or shiitake), sliced
- 1 bell pepper, thinly sliced
- 1 onion, thinly sliced
- 2 cloves garlic, minced
- 1 tablespoon ginger, minced
- 2 tablespoons low-sodium soy sauce or tamari
- 1 tablespoon rice vinegar
- 1 tablespoon hoisin sauce
- 1 tablespoon sesame oil
- 2 tablespoons vegetable oil, divided
- Salt and pepper to taste
- Cooked brown rice or quinoa, for serving
- Optional toppings: sliced green onions, sesame seeds

- Press the block of tofu between two layers of paper towels, weighted down with a couple of large cans, for about 15 minutes to remove excess water. Then, cut the tofu into cubes.

- In a small bowl, whisk together the soy sauce or tamari, rice vinegar, hoisin sauce, and sesame oil to make the sauce. Set aside.

- Heat 1 tablespoon of vegetable oil in a large skillet or wok over medium-high heat. Add the tofu cubes and cook until golden brown on all sides, about 5-7 minutes. Remove the tofu from the skillet and set aside.

- In the same skillet, add the remaining tablespoon of vegetable oil. Add the sliced mushrooms and cook until they release their moisture and start to brown, about 5 minutes.

- Add the bell pepper, onion, garlic, and ginger to the skillet. Stir-fry for another 3-4 minutes until the vegetables are tender-crisp.

- Return the cooked tofu to the skillet and pour the sauce over the tofu and vegetables. Stir well to coat everything evenly. Cook for an additional 2-3 minutes until heated through.

- Season with salt and pepper to taste.

- Serve the tofu and mushroom stir-fry hot over cooked brown rice or quinoa.

- Garnish with sliced green onions and sesame seeds if desired.

Nutritional Information

Calories	300-400 kcal per serving
Protein	20-25 grams
Carbohydrates	30-40 grams
Fat	10-15 grams
Fiber	3-5 grams
Sodium	300-500 milligrams

Baked Fish Tacos with Avocado

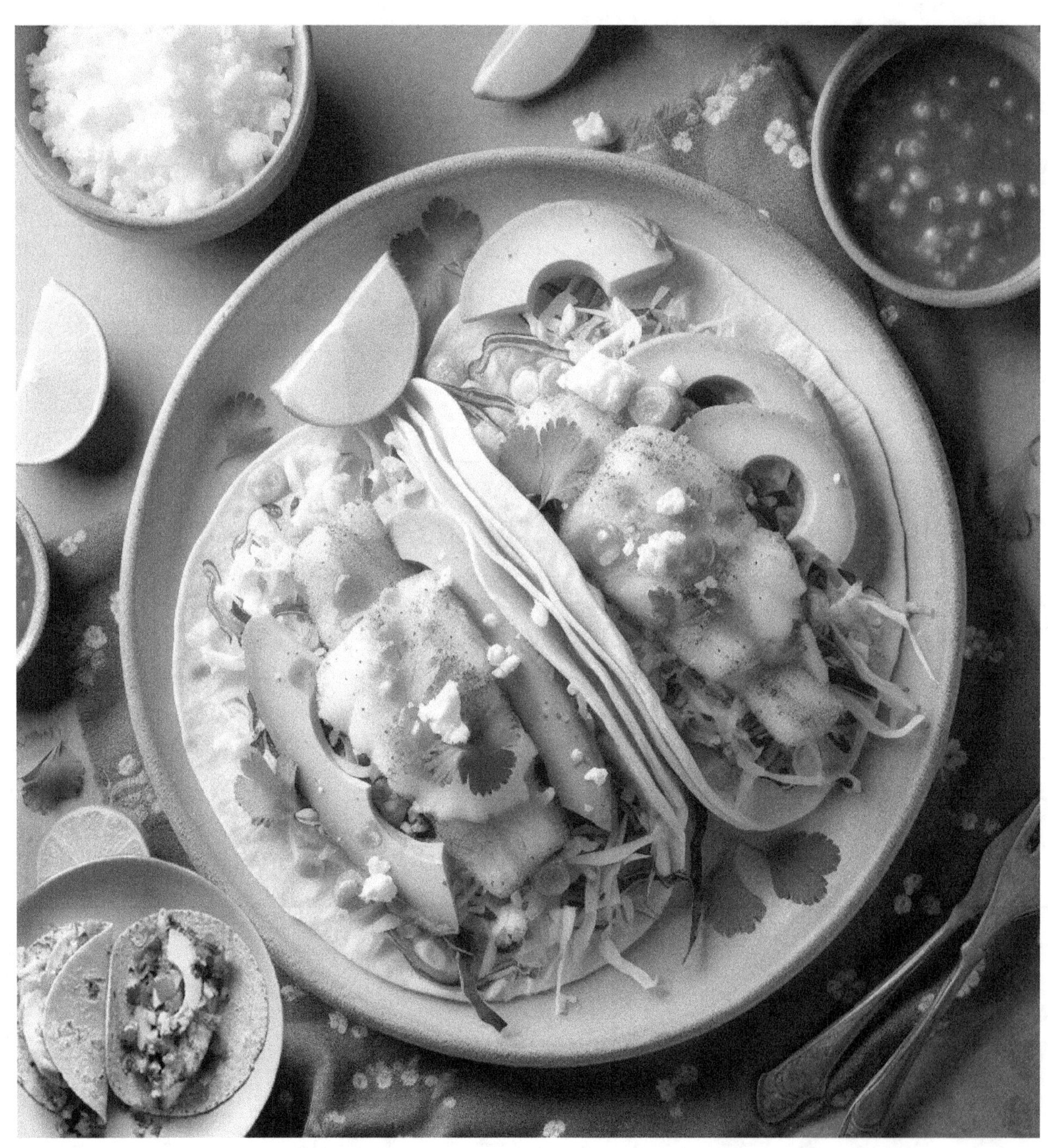

These Fish Tacos are irresistible – they may even win over those who aren't seafood fans! Tender and flaky fish, seasoned to perfection, is nestled on corn tortillas with an array of tasty taco toppings. The crowning touches? A creamy and flavorful fish taco sauce. Easy to prepare yet impressively delicious, these tacos are guaranteed to be a hit every time.

Let me tell you what you are eating in this recipe, Firstly, fish is rich in omega-3 fatty acids, which have been shown to have anti-inflammatory properties and may help reduce the risk of heart disease. Then, there's the avocado, which is like a little green powerhouse of nutrients. It's packed with heart-healthy monounsaturated fats that can help lower bad cholesterol levels and support overall cardiovascular health. Plus, avocados are a fantastic source of potassium, a mineral that plays a crucial role in regulating blood pressure and heart rhythm.

Now, when we talk about the whole grain tortillas, we're talking about fiber. Fiber is your heart's best friend. It helps keep cholesterol levels in check, regulates blood sugar levels, and promotes healthy digestion. By choosing whole grains over refined flour, you're giving your body the fuel it needs to function at its best.

So, when you put it all together, omega-3s from the fish, heart-healthy fats and potassium from the avocado, and fiber from the whole grain tortillas, you've got a meal that not only tastes fantastic but also provides a powerful combination of nutrients

Ingredients:

- 1-pound white fish fillets (such as cod or tilapia)

- 1 tablespoon olive oil

- 1 teaspoon chili powder

- 1 teaspoon ground cumin

- 1/2 teaspoon garlic powder

- 1/2 teaspoon smoked paprika

- Salt and pepper to taste

- 8 small whole grain tortillas

- 1 avocado, sliced

- 1 cup shredded cabbage or lettuce

- 1/4 cup chopped fresh cilantro

- 1 lime, cut into wedges

- Optional toppings: salsa, Greek yogurt or sour cream

Preparation / Direction

- Preheat your oven to 400°F (200°C). Line a baking sheet with parchment paper or lightly grease it with olive oil.

- In a small bowl, mix together the olive oil, chili powder, cumin, garlic powder, smoked paprika, salt, and pepper to create a seasoning blend.

- Pat the fish fillets dry with paper towels, then place them on the prepared baking sheet. Brush both sides of the fillets with the seasoning blend.

- Bake the fish in the preheated oven for 12-15 minutes, or until it flakes easily with a fork.

- While the fish is baking, warm the tortillas according to package instructions.

- Once the fish is cooked, remove it from the oven and use a fork to flake it into bite-sized pieces.

- To assemble the tacos, place a generous portion of the flaked fish onto each tortilla. Top with sliced avocado, shredded cabbage or lettuce, and chopped cilantro. Squeeze fresh lime juice over the top.

- Serve the tacos with additional toppings like salsa, Greek yogurt or sour cream with Avocado

"Cooking is like painting or writing a song. Just as there are only so many notes or colors, there are only so many flavors – it's how you combine them that sets you apart."

_Wolfgang Puck

These recipes are carefully designed with the dietary requirements of those dealing with AFib in consideration. Yet, what sets them apart is their wider appeal and their potential to enhance the well-being of anyone seeking to promote heart health and overall wellness.

_*Lilian Daniel*

As a professional chef deeply committed to the art of culinary creation and the profound impact it can have on our health and well-being, I dedicate this book as message of hope, empowerment, and delicious possibility.

Living with AFib presents unique challenges, there's no denying that. From managing symptoms to making dietary choices that support heart health, the journey can sometimes feel daunting. But let me assure you, dear friends, that in the realm of the kitchen lies a world of opportunity, a world where each chop of the knife, each sizzle of the pan, and each delightful aroma wafting through the air is an act of self-care and nourishment.

Cooking, my friends, is not merely a task to be checked off a list. It is an act of love, an expression of creativity, and a pathway to wellness. When we engage in the sacred art of cooking, we take control of our health in a profound and meaningful way. We choose the ingredients that nourish our bodies, the flavors that delight our senses, and the techniques that elevate simple ingredients into culinary masterpieces.

For those of us navigating the waters of AFib, cooking offers a beacon of hope, a tangible way to support our heart health and improve our overall well-being. With each nutritious meal we prepare, we fortify our bodies with the vitamins, minerals, and antioxidants they need to thrive. We craft dishes that are not only delicious but also tailored to our unique dietary needs, ensuring that every bite brings us one step closer to optimal health.

But let us not forget the joy that cooking brings to our lives. In the kitchen, we find solace, inspiration, and a sense of accomplishment. We bond with loved ones over shared meals, create memories that last a lifetime, and discover the profound connection between food and happiness.

Together, let us find a way that promises not only better health but also greater happiness, fulfillment, and connection. For in the kitchen, miracles happen, one delicious dish at a time.

Recipes to try at Home

1. **Quinoa Salad with Roasted Vegetables and Lemon-Tahini Dressing**

This hearty salad combines protein-rich quinoa with a colorful array of roasted vegetables like bell peppers, zucchini, and cherry tomatoes. The lemon-tahini dressing adds a zesty kick and a dose of heart-healthy fats.

2. **Salmon and Asparagus Foil Packets**

These easy-to-make foil packets are bursting with flavor and nutrition. Fresh salmon fillets are paired with tender asparagus spears and seasoned with herbs, lemon, and a drizzle of olive oil. Simply wrap them up and bake for a delicious and heart-healthy meal.

3. **Mango Avocado Black Bean Salad**

This vibrant salad features a medley of fresh mango, creamy avocado, and protein-packed black beans, all tossed in a zesty lime-cilantro dressing. It's a refreshing and satisfying dish that's perfect for warm weather.

4. Spinach and Feta Stuffed Chicken Breast

Tender chicken breasts are filled with a flavorful mixture of sautéed spinach, tangy feta cheese, and aromatic garlic. Baked to perfection, this dish is packed with protein and essential nutrients to support heart health.

5. Lentil Vegetable Soup

Warm up with a comforting bowl of lentil vegetable soup. Loaded with fiber-rich lentils, hearty vegetables like carrots, celery, and tomatoes, and fragrant herbs and spices, this nourishing soup is both satisfying and nutritious.

6. Grilled Shrimp Skewers with Pineapple Salsa

These grilled shrimp skewers are bursting with tropical flavors! Marinated shrimp are threaded onto skewers, grilled to perfection, and served with a vibrant pineapple salsa. It's a light and refreshing dish that's perfect for summer.

7. Roasted Beet and Goat Cheese Salad

Earthy roasted beets are paired with creamy goat cheese, crunchy walnuts, and tender baby spinach in this elegant salad. A simple balsamic vinaigrette ties everything together for a dish that's as beautiful as it is delicious.

8. Turkey and Vegetable Stir-Fry

Lean ground turkey is stir-fried with an assortment of colorful vegetables like bell peppers, broccoli, and snap peas in this quick and easy dish. Seasoned with ginger, garlic, and soy sauce, it's a flavorful and nutritious meal that comes together in minutes.

9. Stuffed Bell Peppers with Quinoa and Turkey

Bell peppers are filled with a hearty mixture of quinoa, lean ground turkey, diced tomatoes, and spices, then baked until tender. These stuffed peppers are not only delicious but also packed with protein, fiber, and essential nutrients.

10. Greek Yogurt Parfait with Berries and Almonds

Start your day on a nutritious note with a Greek yogurt parfait layered with fresh berries, crunchy almonds, and a drizzle of honey. Greek yogurt is rich in protein and probiotics, while berries and almonds add a dose of antioxidants and healthy fats.

11. Cauliflower Rice Stir-Fry with Tofu

Replace traditional rice with cauliflower rice in this flavorful stir-fry recipe. Tofu adds protein while colorful vegetables like bell peppers, carrots, and snap peas provide vitamins and minerals. Season with soy sauce and ginger for a delicious Asian-inspired dish.

12.   Mediterranean Stuffed Portobello Mushrooms

Portobello mushrooms are filled with a mixture of quinoa, spinach, sun-dried tomatoes, olives, and feta cheese, then baked until tender. These stuffed mushrooms are packed with flavor and nutrients, making them a satisfying vegetarian option.

13.   Baked Chicken Parmesan with Whole Wheat Pasta

Lightly breaded chicken breasts are topped with marinara sauce and melted mozzarella cheese, then served over whole wheat pasta. This healthier version of a classic Italian dish is lower in saturated fat and higher in fiber, making it heart-friendly.

14.   Sesame Ginger Salmon with Stir-Fried Vegetables

Marinate salmon fillets in a mixture of sesame oil, ginger, garlic, and soy sauce, then grill or bake until flaky. Serve with a side of stir-fried vegetables like bok choy, broccoli, and snow peas for a nutritious and flavorful meal.

15.   Chia Seed Pudding with Mixed Berries

Make a creamy chia seed pudding by soaking chia seeds in almond milk or coconut milk overnight, then sweetening with a touch of honey or maple syrup. Serve topped with mixed berries for a nutritious and satisfying breakfast or dessert option.

16. Turkey and White Bean Chili

Lean ground turkey and white beans are simmered in a flavorful broth with tomatoes, onions, peppers, and spices to create a hearty and nutritious chili. Top with a dollop of Greek yogurt and fresh cilantro for added flavor.

17. Soba Noodle Salad with Edamame and Peanut Sauce

Cooked soba noodles are tossed with edamame, shredded carrots, red cabbage, and scallions, then dressed in a creamy peanut sauce made with peanut butter, soy sauce, lime juice, and ginger. This colorful and satisfying salad is perfect for lunch or dinner.

18. Grilled Vegetable Skewers with Quinoa

Thread skewers with colorful vegetables like cherry tomatoes, bell peppers, zucchini, and mushrooms, then grill until tender and lightly charred. Serve over a bed of cooked quinoa for a nutritious and delicious vegetarian meal.

19. Lentil and Vegetable Shepherd's Pie

This hearty and comforting dish features a savory filling made with lentils, carrots, celery, onions, and peas, topped with creamy mashed potatoes. Baked until golden and bubbly, this vegetarian shepherd's pie is sure to become a family favorite.

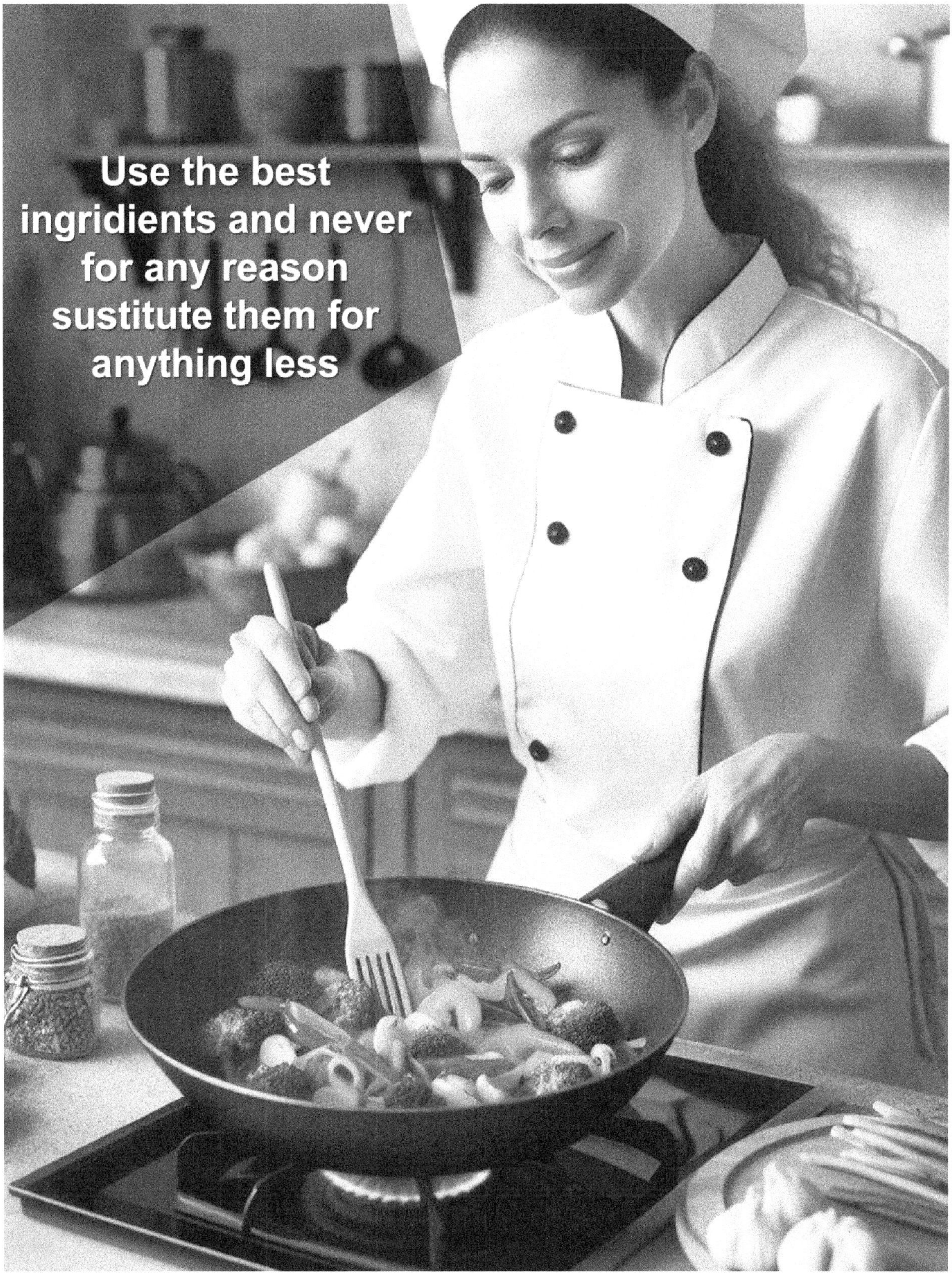

Use the best ingridients and never for any reason sustitute them for anything less
Lilian Daniel